THE BRAIN DRAIN OF HEALTH PROFESSIONALS FROM SUB-SAHARAN AFRICA TO CANADA

Ronald Labonte, Corinne Packer, Nathan Klassen,
Arminee Kazanjian, Lars Apland, Justina Adalikwu,
Jonathan Crush, Tom McIntosh, Ted Schrecker,
Joelle Walker, David Zakus

Series Editor: Prof. Jonathan Crush

African Migration and Development Series No. 2

Acknowledgements

Research was supported through grants from the Canadian Institutes of Health Research and the Saskatchewan Health Research Foundation. David Dorey assisted with editing this report.

Published by Idasa, 6 Spin Street, Church Square, Cape Town, 8001, and Queen's University, Canada.

© Southern African Migration Project (SAMP) 2006
ISBN 1-920118-38-1

First published 2006
Produced by Idasa Publishing

Contents

Tables

Figures

Acronyms

ACHHR	Advisory Committee on Health Human Resources
BC	British Columbia
BMA	British Medical Association
CIC	Citizenship and Immigration Canada
CIHI	Canadian Institute of Health Information
CMA	Canadian Medical Association
CPSO	College of Physicians and Surgeons of Ontario
DENOSA	Democratic Nursing Organisation of South Africa
DFID	Department for International Development
EQUINET	Regional Network for Equity in Health in Southern Africa
GDP	Gross Domestic Product
HHR	Health human resources
HIV/AIDS	Human Immunodeficiency Virus/ Acquired Immunodeficiency Syndrome
HRSDC	Human Resources and Skills Development Canada
ICESCR	International Covenant on Economic, Social and Cultural Rights
IMF	International Monetary Fund
IMG	International Medical Graduate
IOM	International Organisation for Migration
MCC	Medical Council of Canada

MCCEE	Medical Council of Canada Evaluating Examinations
MDG	Millennium Development Goal
MoU	Memorandum of Understanding
NEPAD	New Partnership for Africa's Development
NHS	National Health Service
ODA	Official Development Assistance
OECD	Organisation for Economic Co-operation and Development
PNP	Provincial Nominee Program
RHA	Regional Health Authority
RN	registered nurse
SSA	Sub-Saharan Africa
UK	United Kingdom
USA	United States of America
WHO	World Health Organisation
WTO	World Trade Organisation
WONCA	World Organisation of National Colleges, Academies and Academic Associations of General Practitioners/Family Physicians

1   Introduction

Significant numbers of African-trained health workers migrate every year to developed countries including Canada. They leave severely crippled health systems in a region where life expectancy is only 50 years of age, 16 per cent of children die before their fifth birthday and the HIV/AIDS crisis continues to burgeon.[1] The population of Sub-Saharan Africa (SSA) totals over 660 million, with a ratio of fewer than 13 physicians per 100,000.[2]

SSA has seen a resurgence of various diseases that were thought to be receding, while public health systems remain inadequately staffed. According to one report, the region needs approximately 700,000 physicians to meet the Millennium Development Goals.[3] Understaffing results in stress and increased workloads.[4] Many of the remaining health professionals are ill-motivated, not only because of their workload, but also because they are poorly paid, poorly equipped and have limited career opportunities. These, in turn, lead to a downward spiral where workers migrate, crippling the system, placing greater strain on the remaining workers who themselves seek to migrate out of the poor working conditions.[5] The ultimate result is an incontestable crisis in health human resources throughout SSA, the region suffering most from the brain drain of health care professionals.[6] The situation in SSA has become severe enough that the final report of the Joint Learning Initiative on Human Resources for Health – a two-year global initiative sponsored by a number of donors studying various aspects of human resources for health performance – has concluded that the future of global health and development in the 21st century lies in the management of the crisis in human resources for health.[7]

There is a considerable body of literature attesting to the fact that the migration of skilled professionals from developing to developed countries is large and increasing dramatically.[8] While different experts espouse different reasons for the increase, all agree that it is happening.[9] Developing countries are hit hardest by the brain drain as they lose sometimes staggering portions of their college-educated workers to wealthy countries which can better weather their relatively smaller losses of skilled workers.[10] Highly skilled professionals account for 65 per cent of migrants moving to industrialized countries. The International Organization for Migration (IOM) estimates that about 20,000 Africans leave Africa every year to take up employment in industrialized countries. We do not know how many of these are health care professionals (largely because of inadequate systems for gathering such statistics in African countries).[11] The World Health Organization (WHO), however, found that a quarter to two-thirds of health workers interviewed in a recent study expressed an intention to migrate.[12]

Historically, and specific to the SSA context, the brain drain has meant not only the exodus of human capital but financial resources as well, as African health care professionals left countries with their savings and reinvested very little of their foreign earnings back into the region. There is only recent evidence suggesting that, while the numbers of professionals leaving continue to increase, émigrés are slowly reinvesting some of their earnings back into their countries.[13] Other research raises doubts about the value of such reinvestments, however, particularly when they are in the form of remittances that are generally private welfare transfers back to family members and are often used for consumption rather than for savings.[14]

In recognition of the enormous challenge posed by the international migration of health personnel to health systems in developing countries, the World Health Organization has proclaimed 2005-2015 the decade on human resources for health (HRH).[15]

2 Selected SSA Countries Affected by Brain Drain

The Joint Learning Initiative has estimated that an additional one million health workers will be needed over the next decade to deliver basic health interventions in SSA.[16] The 2005 UK Commission for Africa has called for the world's richest nations to provide $7 billion to develop Africa's health infrastructure.[17] The WHO reports that "even countries such as India and the Philippines, which have long encouraged the export of health and other skilled workers because of their return remittances, are increasingly complaining of domestic shortages, especially in the public sector in rural areas."[18]

The overall impact of international recruitment and retention difficulties in SSA source countries is difficult to assess because of the absence of reliable data. However, the summary country profiles below allow us to form a general picture. The figures provided in Table 1 also demonstrate the extent of shortages of physicians and nurses in SSA countries.

Table 1: Practicing Nurses and Physicians and Expenditure on Health in Selected Countries			
	Total of all nurses, density per 100,000	Total expenditure on health as % of GDP (2002)	Total of all physicians, density per 100,000
Developing countries			
Botswana	241 (1991)	6.0%	28 (1999)
Ghana	64 (2002)	5.6%	9 (2002)
Kenya	90 (1995)	4.9%	13 (1995)
Nigeria	66 (1991)	4.7%	26 (2000)
Philippines	442 (2002)	2.9%	116 (2002)
Senegal	22 (1995)	5.1%	7.5 (1995)
South Africa	388 (2001)	8.7%	69 (2001)
Zambia	113 (1995)	5.8%	6.9 (1995)
Developed countries			
Australia	774 (2001)	9.5%	249 (2001)
Canada	1,010 (2000)	9.6%	210 (2000)
France	667 (2001)	9.7%	329 (2001)
Ireland	1,661 (2005)	7.3%	237 (2001)
Netherlands	1,331 (2001)	8.8%	329 (2001)
United Kingdom	497 (1993)	–	166 (1993)
USA	772 (2002)	14.6%	548 (2000)
Source: Derived from WHO country data. Visit: http://www.who.int/countries.			

2.1 Ghana

Vacancy levels in the Ghana Health Service demonstrate a health care system in crisis. In 2002, there was a nearly 50 per cent shortfall in doctors and 57 per cent shortfall in professional nurses.[19] A 2002 Memo by the Director-General of the Ghana Health Service indicated that more Ghanaian doctors worked outside of Ghana than within. The predominant countries of destination of Ghanaian doctors, ranked in order, are the USA, UK, South Africa and Canada. The predominant ranked countries of destination for nurses are UK, USA, Canada and South Africa. One article reported that in the past decade the country has lost 50 per cent of its professional nurses to Canada, the United Kingdom and the USA.[20] Country preference was reported to depend on factors which include ease of registration with a country's professional bodies, as well as additional costs such as exam fees and airline tickets.

Surprisingly, the total number of applications for nursing has risen significantly in Ghana. In one training school alone, for example, the number of qualified applicants rose from 400 in 2003 to 2000 in 2004. Lack of capacity meant that less than 200 qualified applicants obtained admission. Even this modest figure was made possible by the Government of Ghana's efforts to double admissions into nursing school. It is suggested in this report that the rapid rise is due to individuals being increasingly informed about the opportunities and scope for migration. Indeed, "[b]etter qualified women are going into nursing than before, as an investment in leaving the country."[21]

There is no accurate or detailed assessment available of remittances from health workers, though there are signs of nurses returning from abroad to invest in building homes, starting small businesses and providing support for their families in Ghana.

The Nurses and Midwives Council in Ghana has instituted a policy that restrains nurses from obtaining verification of their certificates until they have worked for at least two years in Ghana post-registration. In addition, all health staff trained at government expense are expected to be bonded for an unspecified period (three to five years) or to refund training costs. Bonding has generally been a failure in Ghana as a result of poor compliance and ease of "buying out" the bond.

2.2   South Africa

South Africa is also reportedly in a new and unenviable position. It has traditionally been a country that both sends and receives migrants, but its rate of export of human capital is now far higher than its rate of import.[22]

The South African Medical Association estimated that at least 5,000 South African doctors moved abroad in 2002.[23] According to DENOSA, the largest nursing union in the country, 300 nurses leave South Africa each month.[24] Eileen Brannigan, head of National Nursing Services for Netcare – one of the largest private hospital companies in the country – says that over 25 per cent of the 90,000 registered nurses in South Africa left the country in 2002 alone. According to Brannigan, the South African Nursing Council gets about 300 queries a month from nurses who have registered or who are querying about registration overseas.[25] In May of 2005, the BBC reported the extent to which South Africa's health service has been hit by an exodus of nurses seeking better pay in countries such as the UK and Saudi Arabia. Through DENOSA, nurses went on strike on 2 May 2005 demanding better pay, including a basic uniform allowance of R1,500 (US$ 241).[26]

South Africa's Health Attaché to the IOM has encouraged the use of bilateral arrangements to manage migration of health care workers, using the example of the Memo of Understanding between South Africa and the UK.[27]

As recently as 4 August 2005, South Africa announced it was to take steps to bring home some of the thousands of its health professionals currently work-ing in Western countries, adding that developed countries could no longer rely on poaching health staff from developing countries, accusing the UK, Australia and the USA as the biggest poachers. The plan is to train more health profes-sionals as well as improve working conditions and salaries in South Africa. In this announcement, South Africa indicated that it was looking at signing various bilateral agreements, like the one signed with the United Kingdom, to manage the brain drain at a government-to-government level.[28]

2.3   Zambia[29]

International migration of skilled and highly skilled Zambians increased rapidly over the last 10 years. The health sector is the most affected by the brain drain. A series of recent reports issued by the Ministry of Health shows that the loss of health workers in the public sector is reaching staggering proportions. In 2003, only slightly over half of the medical, nursing and paramedical posts were filled in public health establishments.[30] Another 2003 study conducted by USAID suggests that, out of the more than 600 doctors trained after inde-pendence in 1964, only 50 remain in the country.[31]

Initially the main destinations of Zambian health workers were more advanced countries in the region, such as South Africa, Botswana and Namibia. These countries continue to attract, but growing numbers of health workers are moving directly overseas to Europe, North America, Australia and New Zealand. Hardly any return migration is reported.

Zambia presents an important case for another reason. Its experience in complying with structural adjustment reforms imposed by the World Bank and the International Monetary Fund (IMF) as conditions to receive loans, grants or debt relief has exacerbated its health problems, undoubtedly contributing to its health professional exodus. [32] Its attempts to curb this outflow are also hampered by ongoing conditionalities. For example, the IMF, under its requirements for a medium-term expenditure framework requires Zambia to restrict its government payroll bill to 8 per cent of GDP. To prevent professionals from leaving the country, and to retain desperately needed teachers and health workers, wage packets and supports caused Zambia's payroll to climb to 8.4 per cent of GDP in 2003. As a result, it was suspended from debt-relief in 2003, requiring it to pay US$377 million in debt servicing costs, US$247 million of which actually went back to the IMF. Zambia was reinstated into the debt-relief program in 2004 when a combination of fiscal austerity and export earnings dropped the wage ratio to 7.8 per cent of GDP – but not before the Dutch government donated US$10 million to pay for more teachers in order to keep the wage ratio within IMF-prescribed guidelines.[33]

3   Methodology

Prompted by, and in partnership with a series of African-based studies on the problem, a study of the impact of international recruitment and migration of health care professionals to Canada from SSA countries was undertaken.

Two research methodologies were used for this study. The empirical research consisted of:

(a)   Focus groups conducted at the International Society for Equity in Health conference in Durban, South Africa (June 2004) in which both health professionals who had left SSA and those who had stayed were asked to share the reasons for their choices.

(b)   Interviews with a sample of physicians who had immigrated to the Canadian province of Saskatchewan from SSA.

(c)   Semi-structured interviews conducted with a purposive sample of key Canadian organizations addressing questions related to existing recruit-ment policies and practices; determinants of migration decisions; and feasibility and desirability of policy options. The key informants from these organizations included federal officials, leaders of national asso-ciations of health professionals, leaders of associations and colleges of provincial health professionals as well as officials of provincial health ministries or regional health authorities. In the case of the latter two, a purposive sample of provinces with relatively high percentages of health care professionals from developing countries was selected. Participants were asked open-ended interview questions and prompted to elaborate on responses which could provide further useful information. Fifty-two stakeholder organizations were asked for an interview, of which 25 accepted.

(d)   The entire set of findings from the interviews, together with policy rec-ommendations from African-based researchers reflecting the choices favoured by source countries, were presented in a day-long colloquium held in Ottawa on 14 October 2005. All respondents in the study, as well as other individuals and organizations in stakeholder or decision-making roles, were invited to participate in the colloquium. The goal of this participatory policy workshop was to refine the options that could be advanced to the Canadian government and other policy forums for adop-tion and implementation, and development of a knowledge translation strategy for this purpose. The results are included in this study report.

Second, a literature review supplemented the empirical research for this study, using published and unpublished sources. Three topics were the foci of this review:

1.   The known and potential impact on health professional migration of the liberalization of health services under Mode 4 (movement of persons) of the World Trade Organization's General Agreement on Trade in Services.

2.   The availability, validity, reliability and policy relevance of existing Canadian and international data sources pertinent to all aspects of our study.

3.   Existing studies assessing the push/pull factors for health professional migration, and policy options for managing the flow so that it does not create any net loss for "sending" countries.

4   Foreign Health Professionals in Canada

4.1   Background

The dynamics of international mobility, migration and recruitment of health care professionals are complex. These dynamics include individual choice, motivations and attitudes to career development and the relative status of health workers in different systems. The approach of Canadian federal and provincial governments and medical bodies in managing domestic human health resources and facilitating or attempting to limit the outflow and inflow is also critical, as is the role of recruitment agencies as intermediaries in the process. The tension and overlap in responsibilities between the federal and provincial governments regarding health and immigration further complicate the policy landscape. Against this complex backdrop, the main objectives of this study were to:

- identify the numbers and trends in the inflow of health care workers from developing countries, specifically SSA countries, to Canada;

- summarize the push and pull factors leading to this migration;

- examine the costs and benefits of this migration to Canada and the developing countries affected;

- examine what Canada has done, is in the process of doing, or could do (in comparison to other countries) to reverse or reduce the brain drain from SSA;

- summarize the views of Canadian stakeholder organizations on the gravity of the brain drain of health care professionals from SSA and the policy options to reduce the drain; and

- determine which options would be likely supported or rejected, along with the reasons why, based on interviews with Canadian stakeholder organizations.

It should be noted that the term "health" or "health care" professionals in this study refers only to doctors and nurses. Interview respondents and research did not address other categories of health professionals. This appropriately reflects the reality of health profession migrant profiles with physicians and nurses far outnumbering other professional groups. For instance, nearly 60 per cent of health care professionals entering Canada on a temporary or permanent status in 2003 were specialist physicians and general practitioners, and approximately 23 per cent were registered nurses. Pharmacists, dieticians, optometrists and various forms of therapists made up the small remainder of migrants.[34] Respondents also typically spoke of foreign-trained health professionals in general rather than those specifically from Sub-Saharan Africa. Acquiring data on SSA health care practitioners in Canada was difficult, as existing data is insufficiently detailed to provide a regional- or country-specific picture.

Canada's Health Care System

The Canadian health care system is complex, and its complexity confounds any simple understanding of the causes of its reliance upon foreign-trained health professionals. The federal government regulates immigration policies. It also provides partial financial support for the provision of public health insurance by the country's ten provinces and three territories, under terms that make identifying the relative size of the federal and provincial contributions very difficult and contentious. Taxes and premiums collected by provincial governments comprise by far the largest source of revenue for individual provincial insurance plans. The federal government's only role in providing health services involves services for the military, indigenous populations, and federal prisoners. With this exception, constitutional authority over the delivery of health care, and of education, resides with provincial and territorial governments. Under the Canada Health Act, the federal government imposes a number of requirements on provincial governments, including universality; comprehensiveness (i.e., coverage for all "medically necessary" services), "portability" among provinces, accessibility and public financing. Provinces that fail to meet these requirements are sometimes, although not always, temporarily penalized by a withdrawal of part of the federal portion of cost-sharing. Nevertheless, there is not a single Canadian health care system, but 10 provincial and 3 territorial health care systems. Moreover, all provinces except Ontario have regionalized their health systems, giving considerable authority over health care decision-making, service delivery and recruitment of health professionals to regional health authorities (RHAs). Provincial governments and self-regulating professional bodies, such as provincial colleges of physicians and nurses, are actively involved in policies and resource decisions that affect domestic health human resource planning, but RHAs (and, in Ontario, individual hospital boards) make decisions about how to fill vacant health professional positions. Further complicating the picture, most physicians practice on a fee-for-service basis, even though their fees are fixed under provincial health insurance plans. The universities that train physicians and nurses are an exclusive (and jealously guarded) provincial jurisdiction. Thus, the division of powers between the Canadian federal and provincial governments, and the regionalization of health services within provinces, make it difficult to assign ultimate responsibility for the Canadian health care system's reliance upon foreign-trained professionals, or to determine whether consensus on policy options to reduce this reliance (with particular attention to its costs to source countries) can be developed.

4.2   Physicians

4.2.1   Foreign-trained Physicians from All Source Countries

According to the Canadian Institute of Health Information (CIHI), nearly one-quarter (22.3 per cent) of physicians in Canada today are foreign-trained.[35] The percentage of foreign-trained physicians practicing in Canada has remained generally level over the period 1999-2003, the period for which the most up-to-date statistics are available (see Table 2 below). However, the countries from which they are migrating are changing somewhat and numbers from SSA are increasing (see Table 3).

Table 2: Numbers of Canadian- and Foreign-Trained Physicians Practicing in Canada, 1999-2003					
	1999	2000	2001	2002	2003
Total Physicians	56,914	57,803	58,546	59,412	59,454
Place of M.D. Graduation					
Canada	43,570	44,372	45,018	45,706	45,832
Foreign	13,274 (23%)	13,333 (23%)	13,370 (22.8%)	13,407 (22.5%)	13,286 (22.3%)
Unaccounted Origin	70	98	158	299	336
Source: CIHI, Supply, Distribution and Migration of Physicians 2003, CIHI, Ottawa 2004, p. 42. Available at: http://secure.cihi.ca/cihiweb/dispPage.jsp?cw_page=AR_14_E.					

Table 3: Number of Physicians from Principal SSA Source Countries Practicing in Canada, 1993-2003							
	Sudan	Zambia	Zimbabwe	Ghana	Uganda	Nigeria	South Africa
1993	7	8	13	27	59	39	1,060
1994	7	10	15	28	54	38	1,136
1995	7	9	15	28	57	46	1,139
1996	7	9	15	31	58	49	1,163
1997	7	10	16	30	57	56	1,197
1998	7	10	16	31	57	61	1,318
1999	8	10	16	31	56	69	1,433
2000	11	12	16	33	57	78	1,473
2001	13	14	16	35	58	93	1,628
2002	14	14	17	36	61	117	1,750
2003	15	14	19	36	63	135	1,679

Source: Canadian Institute for Health Information, Southam Medical Database. Statistics gathered at special request of authors and issued by CIHI on 12 August 2005.

Some provinces are more reliant than others on foreign-trained physicians. Quebec has the lowest percentage of foreign-trained physicians at 10.8 per cent. The low percentage is likely due to the fact that Quebec, as a Francophone province, seeks to recruit primarily French-speaking professionals. Saskatchewan has the highest number of foreign-trained professionals at 52.1 per cent, with the next highest being Newfoundland at 41.4 per cent.[36] The provincial breakdown provided in Figure 1 offers a visual attestation of the variations in the number of foreign-trained physicians working in Canadian provinces and territories in 2004.

Even the radical target Canada reportedly set in 1989 – a zero entrance rate for foreign-trained physicians – did not succeed in curbing migration.[37] The Canadian Medical Association recently reported that the proportion of foreign-trained physicians has only declined by 2 per cent since the 1960s in Canada, the decade when the country experienced its peak physician immigration. The Association estimates that nearly 400 foreign-trained physicians arrive in Canada each year with pre-arranged employment and already licensed to practice.[38] Many others seek licensing and employment after arrival.

The majority of foreign-trained graduates practice family medicine, largely outnumbering foreign-trained clinical, laboratory and surgical specialists combined in all but one province.[39] This does not necessarily mean that all are

trained in family medicine, as the greater majority come to Canada with specialized training and experience but are only, or more easily, able to find work
in family medicine.[40] Foreign-trained physicians also are more likely to work in
rural areas of Canada; in 2004, 26.3 per cent of all physicians in rural Canada
were foreign-educated, compared to 21.9 per cent in urban areas.[41]

Figure 1: Percentage of Canadian-Educated and Foreign-Educated Physicians
by Province/Territory, Canada, 2004

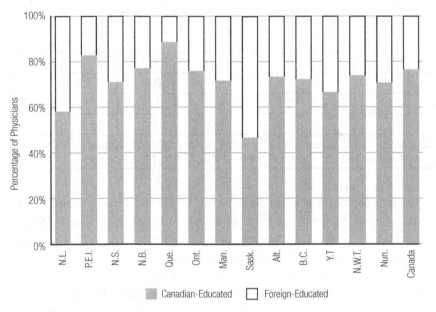

*Source: CIHI, Geographic Distribution of Physicians in Canada: Beyond How Many and
Where, CIHI, Ottawa 2005. Available at: http://secure.cihi.ca/cihiweb/dispPage.jsp?cw_
page=download_form_e&cw_sku=GDPCPDF&cw_ctt=1&cw_dform=N, p. 27.*

Canada is more highly dependent on foreign-trained health care professionals
than most European OECD countries. In Norway, for instance, 13.3 per cent
are foreign-trained while in Belgium the figure is 7.8 per cent and in France
only 3 per cent.[42] A few reasons have been advanced for the comparatively low
number of health professional migrants in European countries. These include
greater admission of foreign students into domestic training programs who
graduate, and are counted, as nationals; socialist traditions resulting in greater
investment in training health care professionals; financial support for studies
such that individuals are not barred from studying nursing and medicine on the
basis of cost; and difficulty in language adaptation in European countries as

opposed to Anglophone countries resulting in fewer migrants going to Europe to work. In contrast, Canada places lower among English-speaking OECD countries; the UK, USA, Australia and New Zealand all have higher proportions of foreign-trained health professionals in their health systems.[43] However, Canada has a comparatively higher proportion of foreign-trained physicians from Sub-Saharan Africa.[44] Of all twelve OECD countries surveyed, Canada had the highest proportion of South African-trained physicians, accounting for nearly 10 per cent of Canada's total population of foreign-trained physicians. The United Kingdom was next with 7 per cent.[45] According to CIHI, between 1986 and 2000 the number of physicians from South Africa alone outnumbered those coming from the UK/Ireland, India and the entire regions of Europe and Asia.[46] On the flipside, six of the twenty countries with the highest emigration factors (arrived at by measuring the loss of physicians from a country as a proportion of the physicians remaining to do the work of health care) are in Sub-Saharan Africa. In declining order these are Ghana, South Africa, Ethiopia, Uganda, Nigeria and Sudan.[47]

4.2.2 Foreign-Trained Physicians from Sub-Saharan African Source Countries

While the number of total foreign-trained physicians practicing in Canada has levelled off in recent years, the number of SSA-trained physicians working in Canada in the last decade has notably increased. In other words, Canada is receiving more and more physicians from the region which can least afford to lose them. While numbers from five of the top SSA source countries have only increased gradually over the last decade, they are increasing nonetheless. Most worrying are the figures from Nigeria and South Africa. Specifically, the number of South African-trained physicians practicing in Canada has risen over 60 per cent in the last 10 years. This is particularly striking because of the sheer numbers at hand: according to the most recent survey, 1,679 South African-trained physicians were practicing in Canada. The number of physicians trained in Nigeria now working in Canada has more than tripled in one decade. Table 3 provides the actual numbers and the year-by-year trends are graphed in Figures 2 and 3.

Figure 2: Number of Physicians from Principal SSA Source Countries Practicing in Canada, 1993-2003

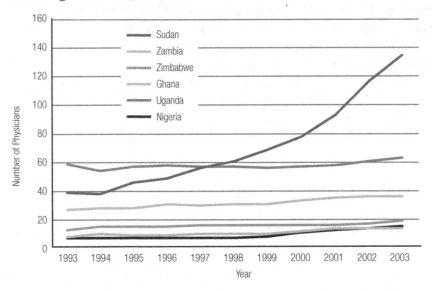

Source: Canadian Institute for Health Information, Southam Medical Database. Statistics gathered at special request of authors and issued by CIHI on 12 August 2005.

Figure 3: Number of South African Physicians Practicing in Canada, 1993-2003

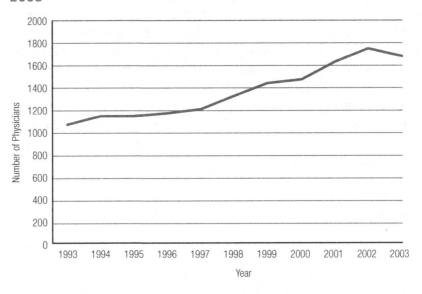

Source: Canadian Institute for Health Information, Southam Medical Database. Statistics gathered at special request of authors and issued by CIHI on 12 August 2005.

An increasing majority of foreign physicians enter Canada on temporary visas.[48] Many enter the country as visa trainees to undertake post-MD training with the expectation that they will return home. Roughly 20 per cent of visa trainees, however, remain in Canada. With this category of visa entry rising (from 779 in 1990 to 1,996 in 2004), the number staying in Canada each year is expected to increase.[49] More research is required into the reasons for this trend and its impact. It would also be wise for Canada to consider the outcome of Australia's decade-old immigration policy to issue more temporary visas to skilled professionals. The policy, described in greater length below, has led to increased numbers of skilled professionals migrating and working in Australia, with a significant proportion eventually changing their temporary status to a permanent one.

Table 4 demonstrates an apparent tendency of foreign-trained physicians in Canada to locate (or be located) as cohorts with members of their own community, ethnic background or country. Numerous respondents suggested the tendency for cohort formation can be attributed to classmates, friends and colleagues following those already established in Canada. It is also likely, however, that recruiters contribute to this formation, hiring graduates from certain SSA universities or hospitals which they believe produce highly qualified physicians. This has been reported in the United States which reportedly recruits the overwhelming majority of SSA-trained physicians.[50]

Another group of physicians typically ignored but worthy of some consideration are those who obtain all or a portion of their training in Canada. There has been a steady increase in the number of foreign-trained physicians completing Canadian residencies funded by Health Canada (the Canadian federal health ministry). From 2003-2004 to 2004-2005 alone, this figure jumped from 591 to 775.[51] There are also a number of foreign-trained physicians completing Canadian residencies who are supported by funds from outside Health Canada, mainly from foreign government contracts. That number jumped from 474 in 1994-1995 to 924 in 2004-2005.[52] What happens to most of these foreign graduates completing residencies in Canada is relatively unknown. Are they obtaining and accepting positions in Canada? Are they obtaining temporary or permanent visas? Does Canada distinguish between those funded by Health Canada and those who are not?

Table 4: Provincial Breakdown of Canadian Physicians Having Graduated from Specified Sub-Saharan African Countries, 2003						
	Alberta	BC	Manitoba	NB	NFLD	NWT
Cameroon	0	0	0	0	1	0
Congo (Brazzaville)	0	0	0	0	1	0
Ethiopia (Abyssinia)	2	0	0	0	0	0
Ghana	1	1	3	0	3	0
Nigeria	17	7	6	4	21	0
South Africa	373	592	134	8	50	2
Somalia	0	1	0	0	0	0
Sudan	1	1	0	0	0	0
Tanzania	3	0	0	0	0	0
Uganda	7	12	2	0	5	0
Zambia	5	4	0	0	0	0
Zimbabwe	2	8	0	1	1	0
TOTAL	411	626	145	13	82	2

	NS	Nunavut	Ontario	PEI	Quebec	SK	Yukon
Cameroon	0	0	0	0	3	0	0
Congo (Brazzaville)	0	0	0	0	0	2	0
Ethiopia (Abyssinia)	1	0	5	0	0	0	0
Ghana	1	0	21	0	0	6	0
Nigeria	6	0	47	0	1	23	0
South Africa	22	1	336	2	13	266	0
Somalia	0	0	0	0	0	0	0
Sudan	1	0	9	0	0	1	2
Tanzania	0	0	4	0	0	0	0
Uganda	1	0	30	0	0	6	0
Zambia	0	0	2	0	1	1	0
Zimbabwe	0	0	5	0	0	2	0
TOTAL	32	1	459	2	18	307	4

Source: Canadian Institute for Health Information (CIHI), Southam Medical Database. Statistics gathered at special request of authors and issued by CIHI on 12 August 2005.

BC = British Columbia; NB = New Brunswick; NFLD = Newfoundland; NWT = North West Territory; NS = Nova Scotia; PEI = Prince Edward Island; SK = Saskatchewan.

4.3   Nurses

4.3.1.   Foreign-Trained Nurses from All Source Countries

The proportion of foreign-trained nurses in Canada is considerably less than that of foreign-trained physicians, representing 7.4 per cent of the total registered nurses in Canada.[53] The province of British Columbia (BC) has the highest proportion of all foreign-trained nurses, whereas the province of Ontario has the greatest proportion of African-trained nurses. Just over a quarter of foreign-trained nurses working in Canada are educated in the United Kingdom. Nearly another quarter was educated in the Philippines, followed by 9 per cent in the United States and 7 per cent in Hong Kong. In general, the number of foreign-trained nurses in Canada has remained constant over the last five years.[54]

4.3.2   Foreign-Trained Nurses from Sub-Saharan Africa

A survey of employed registered nurses in Canada who had graduated in a SSA country found that such nurses come from only 9 of a total of 53 SSA countries. In 2003, 524 nurses in Canada were trained in SSA, over 25 per cent of these in South Africa. Table 5 and Figure 4 demonstrate the upward trend in the number of SSA-trained registered nurses in the Canadian nursing workforce over the last decade. Only countries with 20 or more nationals are represented in the figure. Ethiopia joined these ranks only in 2003, when 20 of its nurses worked in Canada that year. Like their physician counterparts, South African nurses represent the overwhelming majority of SSA-trained nurses now practicing in Canada, with nearly three times more nurses than the next most represented group from Nigeria. As with their physicians counterparts, the large increase in Nigerian-trained nurses practicing in Canada (from 0 to 67 over one decade) is also noteworthy.

Table 5: Number of RNs from Principal SSA Source Countries Practicing in Canada, 1993-2003					
	Ghana	Kenya	Nigeria	Senegal	South Africa
1993	23	40	0	44	109
1994	21	40	10	46	108
1995	22	24	13	30	82
1996	29	39	18	18	129
1997	22	24	19	36	93
1998	24	48	24	37	127
1999	32	45	30	40	127
2000	33	41	31	37	128
2001	34	38	41	36	151
2002	42	36	49	37	169
2003	53	47	67	39	195

Source: Canadian Institute for Health Information (CIHI), Southam Medical Database.
Statistics gathered at special request of authors and issued by CIHI on 12 August 2005.

Figure 4: Number of RNs from Principal SSA Source Countries Practicing in Canada, 1993-2003

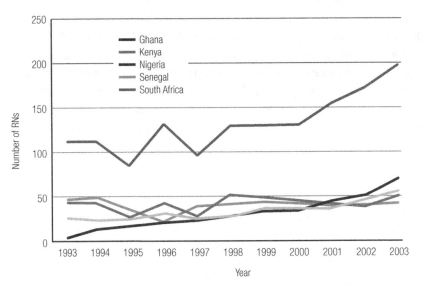

Source: Canadian Institute for Health Information (CIHI), Southam Medical Database.
Statistics gathered at special request of authors and issued by CIHI on 12 August 2005.

Table 6 shows the distribution of SSA-trained nurses in Canada in 2003. Only provinces with five or more SSA-trained nurses are listed. The table suggests that nurses from specific countries tend to congregate in the same provinces. With the exception of Senegalese-trained nurses congregating in Quebec for obvious linguistic reasons, it is not possible to establish whether this phenomenon is the result of targeted recruitment by provinces or of simple word-of-mouth from nationals based in Canada. No nursing colleges and associations interviewed claimed knowledge of active or targeted recruitment, lending plausibility, though not certainty, to the latter hypothesis of nurses self-locating.

Table 6: Number of Employed Registered Nurses by African Graduation and Province, 2003*

	QUE	ONT	MAN	SASK	ALTA	BC
Dem. Rep. of Congo	9	5				
Zimbabwe		7				
Ethiopia		22				
Ghana		47				6
Kenya		24			11	12
Nigeria		42				7
Senegal	39					
Somalia		11				
South Africa		76	8	11	21	79
Total*	67	256	18	18	42	112

* Including nurses from SSA countries with fewer than 5 nurses in any province or territory

Source: Canadian Institute for Health Information, Registered Nurses Database. Statistics gathered at special request of authors and issued by CIHI on 12 August 2005.

4.4 Reasons for Migration

Even if active and passive recruitment were completely done away with (thus abolishing a pull factor), health professionals from all countries would probably still migrate to Canada. Health professionals from developing countries, in particular, would still be driven to migrate because of strong push factors. Most respondents in this study felt that, in order to diminish the large numbers of migrant health professionals, source countries had to deal with their push factors. There was general consensus that there would always be "natural mobility" – people moving to new countries without being either "pushed" or "pulled." Others added that health care professionals are typically mobile by nature and are more likely to move from place to place following jobs. Nearly all respondents commented that significant numbers of foreign physicians and nurses come to Canada because they are encouraged by family members, old friends, colleagues and schoolmates who have already moved and are working in Canada. All respondents felt that no organizations or employers in Canada were actively recruiting foreign-trained health care professionals at this time. Such recruitment certainly has taken place in the past. Whether or not "active recruitment" is still occurring remains a moot point. Importantly, however, respondents noted that new modes of recruitment fell within a grey zone of "passive recruitment."

Finally, numerous respondents stressed that Canada was not the clear winner in the migration cycle; the freedom to seek migration also means that foreign- and Canadian-trained health professionals subsidized by Canadian funds are free to emigrate. Data on the numbers of physicians who have left and returned to Canada from 1992-2003 reveals that Canada does experience a net loss of physicians. However, this loss is not as great as some might believe, totalling 3,838 physicians over a period of 11 years.

4.4.1   Push and Pull Factors of Migration

The brain drain is triggered in part by pull (demands for skilled labour in more advanced and industrialized countries) as well as push factors (difficulties encountered in source developing countries including negative effects of structural adjustment programs on health systems).[55] A number of respondents felt quite strongly that it is not so much pull as push factors that are influencing health professionals to leave their countries: more must be done in SSA and other source countries to eliminate the push factors. Few of the organizations felt it was their duty or within their mandate to address push factors. Most felt these matters should be addressed at a different level (e.g. by the World Bank or by the Canadian International Development Agency); brain drain was therefore largely out of their control and, in many instances, not a priority for their organization.

Respondents spoke of the difficult situations faced by many health care professionals in source countries. They are in a giving and caring profession and, for the most part, are committed individuals. In the end, however, they also need money to survive and often simply do not earn enough in the countries they leave. Sometimes migration is intended to be a short-term affair to pay off medical debts in the source country. As one foreign-trained physician working in Canada commented: "We came to Canada with a view of paying off debt and to getting a chance to travel, so it was really, basically to earn enough money to pay off medical school fees that accrued during training." Respondents also emphasized the frustration permeating the profession. Despite their training, they are unable in their developing countries to provide even the most basic health care. In short, they are unable to practice what they have been trained to do.

One respondent noted that, specific to South Africa, there is an overarching concern with personal security that is also racialized. Health care providers coming to Canada sense an opportunity to live and work in a country that does not have the same degree of social instability and racial tension.

A number of female respondents made mention of gender-specific push factors. These ranged from poorer pay and working conditions in the health care professions, nursing in particular, to safety concerns on and off the job, including decisions not to work late into nightfall because of risk of aggression while returning home, particularly in rural areas.

Respondents frequently cited the threat of HIV infection as another push factor for health care practitioners from SSA, particularly from South Africa. A recent article on health human resource (HHR) strategy in the region reports that the crisis in SSA is partially a result of the significant burden of HIV/AIDS. HIV/AIDS, it reports, "represents a special cause of wastage in Africa. Deaths of health workers, fear of infection, burnout, absenteeism, heavy workloads and stress affect productivity."[56] In its ambitious Action Plan to Prevent Brain Drain, Physicians for Human Rights summarizes findings that the fear of occupational infection is a significant reason why health care workers are emigrating. Fear of contracting HIV was specifically cited as a push factor in Malawi, Zambia and Zimbabwe.[57] The Regional Network for Equity in Health in Southern Africa (EQUINET) further reports that the perception that nursing is a high-risk profession is proving a deterrent to potential applicants. According to the EQUINET report, the HIV seroconversion risk among surgeons in tropical Africa may be 15 times higher than in developed countries. A study in one South African hospital found that 63.1 per cent of nurses had experienced accidental blood exposure and 49.5 per cent had experienced a needlestick injury.[58] The annual occupational risk of HIV transmission was estimated at 0.27 per cent for health workers. Among surgeons, the risk was 0.7 per cent (i.e. more than twice as high) if no special protective measures were taken. As a result, staff become infected, fall ill, and die. If the disease progresses rapidly, this results in sudden vacancies with little time to plan recruitment; if slowly, staff may be on long-term indefinite sick leave with no indication of when or whether they may return. Both scenarios present difficulties for health human resources planning and management.[59]

Country-specific surveys on the migration of health professionals similarly demonstrate common and multiple factors for the decision to emigrate. For instance, a WHO study of five SSA countries found all respondents cited four general factors, but the primary reason was "better/more realistic remuneration."[60] A SAMP survey of the South African brain drain found that factors for emigration also varied according to the age group of health professionals.[61]

On the pull side, respondents described how passive, rather than active, recruitment plays a role in getting health professionals to come to Canada. Sources of passive recruitment are much more difficult to control and largely considered an inevitable outcome of the global and electronic age. Aside from passive recruitment, Canada's positive characteristics (wealth, safety, education) were thought to attract foreign health care professionals to the country.

A recent study on the reasons physicians migrate to developed countries echoes the reasons listed by our stakeholders. Although responses varied somewhat according to the country surveyed, a desire for increased income, greater access to enhanced technology, an atmosphere of general security and stability, and improved prospects for one's children were the primary motivating factors for physician migration.[62] Specific to South Africa, SAMP's study of motivations for migration of South African health care professionals and trainees reemphasizes these reasons, although peculiarities of the historical and political context of the country led respondents to stress safety and personal security.[63]

In 2004, South Africa's Health Attaché, speaking at the IOM, recognized numerous push factors for South African health care professionals, notably: economic (perceived level of salaries and exchange rates); political (perceived crime rate, perceived economic security and a general uncertainty about the future); and job related (conditions of service; overworking, understaffing, lack of opportunities for professional growth and development and an environment not conducive for productivity). She also referred to numerous pull factors, notably economic (desire to improve financial status and build a nest egg, aggressive recruitment, tax exemptions and ability to settle debts); social (including personal security and stability and better educational opportunities for children); and career opportunities.[64]

According to the Democratic Nursing Organisation of South Africa (DENOSA), South African nurses cited working conditions as the principal push factor. One nurse explains: "I never thought I would be one of the nurses leaving. I criticized many of my colleagues when they left. Then I found that, as nurses were leaving, those of us who were left had to carry the load. In my hospital… there were about 500 outpatients a day and only 14 to 15 nurses allocated to this section. How can we give good care in these conditions?" The Deputy Director of DENOSA agrees that South African nurses are generally frustrated with their pay, long shifts, conditions of work and treatment.

4.5 Active and Passive Recruitment

All respondents from Canadian stakeholder organizations acknowledged the important contribution of foreign-trained health professionals to the Canadian health care system. Most stressed that, despite the absence of explicit statements on international recruitment by most of their organizations, the general understanding and modus operandi of their organizations is that active recruitment of health professionals from developing countries, in particular SSA, is unethical and not to be condoned. A number of organizations made reference to the Commonwealth Code of Practice on the International Recruitment of Health Professionals and its guiding principles. Another organization, the World Organization of National Colleges, Academies and Academic Associations of General Practitioners/Family Physicians (WONCA), drafted and signed on to a collaborative instrument – the Code of Practice for the International Recruitment of Health Care Professionals, referred to as "The Melbourne Manifesto" – which discourages recruitment from developing countries. Only one respondent referred to the Manifesto. Aside from endorsing or claiming support for these codes, no stakeholder organization interviewed had adopted its own explicit policies against the active recruitment of foreign-trained health care workers.

Most respondents stressed that, barring a few exceptions in the recent past, Canada has not engaged in active recruitment. The few incidents of active recruitment that had occurred (e.g. when the government of the province of Alberta went on a recruitment mission to South Africa to hire physicians because of a severe provincial shortage) were cited as real exceptions. These were largely frowned upon as unethical while being excused as desperate actions to resolve desperate situations, although without consideration given to the health impact on source countries.

Whereas the occurrence of active recruitment was fervently dismissed, respondents noted the delicate line between active and passive recruitment. As one respondent explained: "We've created a situation where we no longer have to actively recruit because of digital communications, the [reach of] medical or health journals… and the kind of secondary market of private recruiters." The resulting effect is that "we're slowly removing barriers to people" who may wish to migrate.

One respondent also remarked that the failure of countries like Canada to properly plan its health human resources "creates a situation where even so-called passive recruitment or even the seeking of migration becomes a de facto form of active recruitment." The basic logic advanced was that if there were considerably fewer positions for health professionals in Canada there would likely be fewer foreign-trained health professionals seeking to migrate to Canada.

4.6 Government Measures Bolstering Passive Recruitment

Measures taken by the federal and provincial governments are further bolstering passive recruitment. They include:

4.6.1 Evaluating Exams in Foreign Countries

The Medical Council of Canada (MCC), responsible for licensing physicians to practice in Canada, has developed off-shore Evaluating Exams (MCCEE). In 2005, exams could be taken in eight countries, although none are operating in SSA. A new evaluation centre in New Delhi, India, was confirmed in 2005. Applications for the New Delhi centre are accepted on a first-come, first-served, space availability basis.[65] Such measures were largely welcomed by respondents since individuals thinking of immigrating would know whether they would be licensed in Canada and could make a better informed decision. Respondents considered these measures as a means to reduce "brain waste" (the image of foreign-trained physicians working as taxi drivers in Canada) as well as decrease "brain drain" (at least insofar as health professionals facing licensure difficulties may be less inclined to consider seeking migration to Canada). At the same time, respondents recognized that, while this did not constitute active recruitment it actively removed barriers resulting in a de facto recruitment system. That being said, the current fee for the MCCEE ($1000) as well as additional costs incurred in preparing for the exams is prohibitive for many candidates.[66] Further, the time required to prepare for this exam is significant and impacts on an individual's earning capacity during this period. Consequently, many candidates abandon the process because of financial limitations.

In 2005 the Medical Council of Canada took another step which ultimately facilitates the employment of foreign-trained physicians in Canada. All United States medical graduates and physicians who have obtained their specialty training in a US postgraduate program are now exempt from the requirement of the Evaluating Examination. As a result, the BC College of Physicians and Surgeons' Registration Committee alone reports that it has seen a "substantial increase in the number of applications from American graduates and International Medical Graduates (IMGs) from the United States."[67]

4.6.2   A New Points System for Immigrants

Until recently, individuals seeking to immigrate to Canada were considered against an "occupation list" defined by Citizenship and Immigration Canada (CIC) which prioritized the types of professionals needed by Canada. If their profession appeared on this list their immigration would be prioritized. Neither physicians nor nurses appeared on this priority list. On 28 June 2002, CIC replaced the "occupation list" system with a new points system for immigrants where individuals with advanced years of academic training gain more points and thereby gain entry more easily. The new system, which reflects Canada's immigration policy, has an inherent bias towards skilled and experienced professionals. By virtue of years of training for physicians (degrees and years of training are the criteria for the education category), this grading system automatically places health professionals near the top of the immigration list. Table 7 illustrates the points system. It is not difficult to see how a 41-year-old physician, speaking English or French, with 15 years of practice and a job offer from a Canadian health authority or hospital would reach the 67 points needed to be accepted.

Table 7: Canadian Immigration and Customs Points System		
1. Education	Maximum	25 Points
2. Official languages	Maximum	24 Points
3. Experience	Maximum	21 Points
4. Arranged Employment	Maximum	10 Points
5. Age (21 – 49)	Maximum	10 Points
6. Adaptability	Maximum	10 Points
TOTAL POINTS	Maximum	100 Points
Source: Citizenship and Immigration Canada. Available at: http://www.cic.gc.ca/english/ skilled/qual-5.html.		

The category of "Skilled Worker" (into which health care professionals fall) is the one most commonly used by applicants from all over the world, and accounts for over 60 per cent of all Canadian immigrants. The Canadian Medical Association (CMA) estimates that an average of 400 foreign-trained health care professionals arrive in Canada each year with pre-arranged employment, and licensed to practice.[68] Information on how many of these are from SSA is not readily available.

4.6.3   Provincial Nominee Programs

The Provincial Nominee Program (PNP) is a program that has been negotiated between nine of Canada's provinces and the federal government to help the provinces address strategic skill shortages. Manitoba was the first province to enter into this agreement, in 1996.[69] The program varies slightly between provinces but in essence it is an agreement that allows individual provinces to nominate individuals to the federal government for landed immigrant status.[70] It is important to note that, in most provinces, foreign-trained health professionals and other skilled professionals falling within the program can only be nominated when it has been shown that a position cannot otherwise be filled by a Canadian. Thus, in approving a nomination, the Canadian Government is accepting the argument that there is an absence of an equally-skilled Canadian-trained health professional.

Shortages in health care professionals exist within each province, but some provinces (notably British Columbia and Saskatchewan) have implemented a special stream of the PNP specifically for medical professionals. Table 8 shows that significant numbers of skilled professionals have entered through this program, particularly in provinces which receive large numbers of foreign-trained health care professionals.

All nominees must already have a valid job offer within the province. The PNP therefore encounters physicians or nurses after they have been recruited but before they have received landed immigrant status. Before applying to immigrate to Canada, potential Provincial Nominees must complete the provincial nomination process. After they have been nominated by a province, they have to make a separate application to Citizenship and Immigration Canada (CIC) for permanent residence. A CIC officer will then assess their application based on Canadian immigration regulations. Provincial Nominees are not assessed on the six selection factors of the Federal points system. Rather, they are in a special stream of their own.

In a pilot project within Saskatchewan conducted with the Regina-Qu'Appelle Health Authority, "[nominated applicants] generally attain their landed immigrant status in a much shorter length of time than through the usual immigration processes."[71] Since the PNP significantly speeds up this process it is not unreasonable to assume that individual hospital boards or regional health authorities will make (or have already made) use of this mechanism to facilitate the immigration of health workers considered in short domestic supply.

As the program is new there is relatively little data on the employment categories of individuals who come through it, and none at all currently available on their country of origin. However, at least one province has stated it specifically entered into the PNP agreement to address its shortage of health workers. British Columbia's program was implemented in March 2001. The initial focus was to mitigate the shortage of Registered Nurses in B.C.[72] Importantly, the PNP provides an expedited pathway to permanent status for foreign health care professionals. According to the BC College of Physicians and Surgeons, once an application has been received, permanent residency should be provided within six to nine months. Previously, many physicians encountered delays of up to three years in obtaining landed status.[73] Health Match BC, an organization funded by the British Columbia department of health, ensures provincial nominees within the health stream are qualified to practice within the province. Table 7 shows that British Columbia has grown to be the second most active province in employing the provincial nominee program.

Table 8: Intake of Nominees for All Provinces with Provincial Nominee Programs

	2000	2001	2002	2003	2004	Total
Newfoundland	0	35	38	37	171	281
Prince Edward Island	0	0	10	44	141	195
Nova Scotia	0	11	0	0	64	75
New Brunswick	22	71	105	146	161	505
Manitoba	1095	973	1530	3116	4048	10762
Saskatchewan	37	41	73	173	323	647
Alberta	19	19	24	178	426	666
British Columbia	13	24	206	441	598	1282
Total	1186	11[74]	1986	4135	5932	14413

Source: Citizenship and Immigration Canada.
Available at: http://www.cic.gc.ca/english/monitor/issue09/05-overview.html (Table 3).

Raw statistics on the composition of British Columbia's inflow of workers were unavailable, but a bar chart acquired from the province's Statistics Department indicates that 25-30 per cent of British Columbian provincial nominees are health care workers. 74 Of the 598 provincial nominees who entered into British Columbia in 2004, 150-170 were health care workers, of which 28 were nurses.[75] The number of the remaining health care workers who were physicians is unknown.

Saskatchewan, a Canadian province with a low population and significant physician retention problems, has been increasing its use of the PNP each year. Although no statistics are available, press releases from the Saskatchewan government indicate that "since expanding the program to include a Health Professions category, the province has nominated 17 nurses and 107 doctors from South Africa, Pakistan, India, the Philippines, and elsewhere." The province began nominating physicians in June 2002 and included nurses in September 2003.[76] Based upon available gross statistics, this indicates that 22 per cent of all nominees since 2002 have been physicians or nurses. Recruitment of South African physicians in Saskatchewan does not seem to be decreasing.[77] Information from CIHI and job advertisements in South African journals corroborated this observation.[78] It appears that the recruitment of South African medical professionals is ongoing across Canada and may have even intensified since the late 1990s, although there is also an obvious need for more detailed and accurate data on these trends, and the role played by the PNP.

Manitoba is by far the most active province with regards to the PNP. It was the first to implement a PNP and is almost eight times more active in its nominations than the next most active province. A recent report indicates that 3 per cent of provincial nominees in Manitoba in 2004 were health workers.[79]

Figure 5: The Provincial Nominee Program

Source: Citizenship and Immigration Canada. Available at: http://www.cic.gc.ca/english/mon-

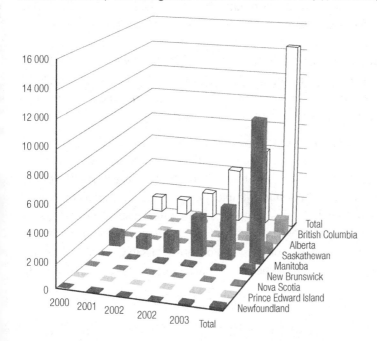

itor/issue09/05-overview.html (Table 3).

Initial research indicates that provincial health ministers were aware of recruitment from South Africa when the PNPs were negotiated and that various members of the legislative assembly applauded the recruitment, as it addressed physician shortages within the communities they represented. At the very least, given statements on government websites, it is clear that provincial governments see the PNP as a means to address physician and nurse shortages. As one example, the Government of Nova Scotia reports:

The Nova Scotia Nominee Program has been developed to assist the Department of Health and District Health Authorities in filling critical shortages in the workforce (this is a special component of the Canadian immigration program). This program should help expedite the immigration process for licensable international medical graduates able to work in Nova Scotia.[80]

4.6.4   Recently Announced Government Pledges

On 25 April 2005, the Canadian federal government announced that it would set aside $75 million to be spent on initiatives to facilitate the migration and employment of foreign health care professionals. Among the initiatives was creation of a national agency to bring more foreign-trained physicians and other medical professionals to Canada. Other initiatives were to establish a national agency to verify credentials of foreign-trained physicians, a website to help foreign-trained physicians prepare to become licensed, and a database to track their progress.[81]

On 18 October 2005, (then) Human Resources Minister Belinda Stronach announced the Government's intention to hold a summit to tackle the problem of recognition of foreign credentials that would allow professionals to work in their fields in Canada. The Minister's intention was to look at ways to speed up and to "address better ways to get information to prospective immigrants before they reach Canada."[82] Stronach said the summit would look at ways of putting people in contact with professional organizations in Canada before they immigrate so they can set the wheels in motion to complete the paperwork to get recognition of their skills.[83]

4.7   The Recruiters

Research and interview findings demonstrate that there are a number of different types of recruiters of health care professionals within and outside of Canada. All stakeholder organizations believed they were not actively recruiting foreign-trained health care professionals. Many believed that foreign-trained health care professionals were self-motivated and unassisted when seeking jobs in Canada and emigrating.

4.7.1   Recruitment Agencies

There are a relatively small number of formal "recruitment agencies" in Canada that specialize in health care professionals. Agencies may be partially or entirely government-funded while others are non-profit based. They may also have a focus, such as the placement of physicians in rural areas. The recruitment agencies interviewed stressed that they were not involved in the active recruitment of foreign-trained health care professionals, as they did not specifically target this group. Indeed, none were advertising specifically abroad but would accept individuals already in Canada. While their advertising (typically on websites) could obviously reach audiences in source countries, this was not their intended audience. For these reasons, the agencies qualified their recruitment as "passive."

4.7.2   Regional Health Authorities

Since authority for hiring hospital-based or other salaried health professionals has devolved to regional health authorities (RHAs) in most Canadian provinces, it is logical to assume that they may be actively recruiting candidates for vacant positions from other parts of Canada, or internationally. It is difficult to know precisely what role RHAs may be playing in recruitment of foreign-trained health professionals. However, the careers section of the South African Medical Journal, the leading medical journal in the SSA region, carries dozens of advertisements by Canadian RHAs for physicians to come and work in their regions, usually located in rural British Columbia, Saskatchewan and Alberta.[84] All advertise highly lucrative pay scales and one additionally offers an "excellent employee benefit plan" including "a relocation assistance package, furnished housing, 6 weeks of vacation and 3 weeks of education leave." The advertisements placed in this journal are clearly targeted at physicians from South Africa or the SSA region, presenting an arguably active form of recruitment. This example also serves as evidence that RHAs are recruiting at both ends – in source countries and in Canada through the PNP system in their provinces.

4.7.3   Private Practice Clinics in Canada

While no survey respondent made mention of physicians or groups of physicians in Canada recruiting colleagues from abroad, it appears to be more common than imagined. The same issues of the South African Medical Journal, for instance, have a handful of advertisements placed by small clinics (comprised of no more than five physicians) seeking to recruit physicians or specialists for their clinics. All are based in rural or small cities in BC, Alberta and Saskatchewan.[85]

4.7.4   Recruiters Based in SSA Countries

Numerous respondents also spoke of aggressive recruiters principally based in South Africa, and cited these as a critical factor in encouraging and assisting health care workers to move and in directing them towards certain countries or to certain employers within countries. Respondents explained how such agents – as unofficially appointed head-hunters – regularly contact regional health authorities and hospitals with qualified candidates already willing and able to migrate. As one example, the September 2005 issue of the South African Medical Journal has three recruitment agencies based in South Africa advertising possible jobs in Canada and elsewhere, one claiming a high rate of success obtaining exceptionally lucrative placements abroad for experienced general practitioners, and another offering to conveniently arrange interviews for foreign jobs in South Africa itself.[86]

4.7.5   Individuals as "Recruiters" in Canada

Interview respondents also spoke often and at length of foreign-trained health care workers already in Canada telling friends, colleagues and former classmates about opportunities known to them and encouraging and facilitating migration. For a significant number of respondents this represented the main source of new foreign-trained health care professionals seeking to migrate to Canada. Some reported that spouses of foreign-trained health workers now settled in Canada act as contact and recruiter.

5   Shortages of Health Professionals in Canada

5.1   Physicians[87]

There is a growing consensus that Canada is facing a physician shortage unprecedented since the inception in the early 1970s of Medicare (the name of Canada's single-payer public health insurance system).[88] Growing lists of communities with family physicians not accepting new patients, cancelled surgeries, difficulties staffing emergency departments and waiting lists for specialist services give force to this consensus.[89]

The shortage is likely to exacerbate Canada's need for foreign-trained physicians, should inadequate planning for human resources for health continue. Provincial colleges and associations are not hiding the fact that they are, and will be increasingly, dependent on foreign-trained physicians to prevent health care crises in their provinces. The Ontario Medical Association, for instance, reports that the province needs a minimum of 2,100 physicians and that one of the measures taken to meet this huge demand is to increase certification of those who are trained abroad.[90] The BC College of Physicians and Surgeons, in its 2005 Annual Report, says it will continue to rely on physician immigration in the foreseeable future for the provision of health care to the population of BC.[91] One way in which this is facilitated is through licensing physicians on a temporary register until they obtain the credentials for full licensure.

In the short span of a decade Canada moved from a perceived physician surplus to a perceived physician shortage. In 1991 the landmark Barer-Stoddart report on physician human resources conveyed concerns of a physician surplus in Canada.[92] The report recommended, inter alia, a 10 per cent reduction in medical school positions. This particular recommendation was adopted and the early period of the 1990s saw the start of a decrease in the number of medical student graduates. In 1997-2000 the number of entrants was 9 per cent lower than the 1991-1996 level. Aside from declines in medical school entrants, the late 1990s saw physicians reporting increased dissatisfaction with rising workloads and concern over an exodus of physicians to the United States. Canada was losing both medical school entrants and licensed physicians.

A 2005 report on the state of Canadian health care illustrates how Canada fares in comparison to other OECD countries. In 2002, Canada ranked twenty-fourth out of 27 selected OECD countries in the number of doctors per 1,000 population.[93]

Figure 6: Doctors per 1,000 Population in OECD Countries, 2002

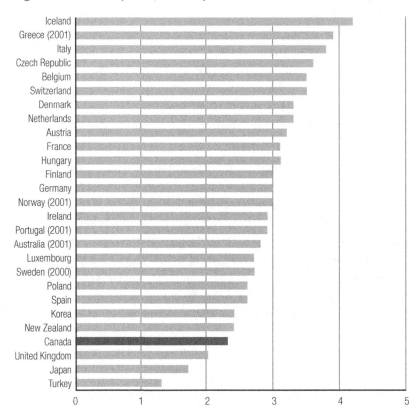

Source: OECD, 2004. Cited and calculated by N. Esmail and M. Walker in How Good is Canadian Health Care? 2005 Report: An International Comparison of Health Care Systems, The Fraser Institute, Vancouver, 2005. Available at: http://www.fraserinstitute.ca/admin/ books/files/HowGoodIsCanHealthCare2005.pdf.

Between 1990 and 2003, the number of doctors per capita remained stable in Canada while it continued to increase at least slightly in most OECD countries.[94] In 2003, Canada had 2.1 practicing physicians per 1,000 population, well below the OECD average of 2.9.

Work published by the Joint Learning Initiative on Human Resources for Health (2004) using WHO health worker data shows statistically that an average of 2.5 trained health workers (nurses, midwives and physicians) per 1,000 population is needed to provide the basic level of access needed to sustain health service delivery in a country.[95] By this account, Canada has a more than adequate supply (physician and nurse density of 11.9/1000) for minimal needs (in contrast to many of the SSA countries from which it receives health professional migrants), although clearly citizen and political expectations are for a Canadian health system that meets more than just a basic level of care.

Canada, like most countries, experiences problems obtaining and retaining physicians in rural areas and the more sparsely populated provinces. The northern regions (Yukon, the Northwest Territories and Nunavut) suffer serious shortages within their vast regions (Table 9). The province of Saskatchewan, despite being proportionately the largest recipient of foreign-trained physicians, has experienced a net decrease in the number of practicing physicians. Manitoba has suffered the same fate. While it is true that the populations of these provinces and territories have only increased slightly over the 2000-2004 period, they have grown nonetheless and were already experiencing shortages in physicians. According to crude projections, the CMA estimates that even if medical school enrolment were increased to 2,500 by the year 2007, Canada would still need over 300 new foreign-trained physicians a year to meet domestic health service delivery demands.[96]

While the ideal route in all provinces is for all physicians to have full licensure for the practice of medicine (meaning they are fully registered for independent practice without restrictions), another route is being widely used. In eight out of ten provinces, some physicians (primarily foreign-trained) are under limited licensure as part of the solution to the health human resource shortage. As the BC College of Physicians and Surgeons reports, "as long as we are dependent on foreign-trained physicians, it will be necessary to continue licensing physicians on the temporary status until they obtain the credentials for full licensure."[97] In BC alone, the ratio of newly registered physicians from South Africa accorded temporary (limited) licensure compared to full licensure in 2005 was more than 2 to 1.[98] Limited licensure, therefore, is one measure used by Canadian licensing bodies to ease foreign-trained physicians into the Canadian job market and thereby meet demand. While it may be true that foreign-trained physicians who quickly gain their full licence to practice in Canada have a greater likelihood of staying to work in Canada, those on limited ("temporary") licences can remain working in Canada on this status for many years before moving on to another country, returning to their countries of origin or eventually obtaining the full licence.

Table 9: Total Number of Physicians in Canada According to Province and Territory, 2000-2004					
	2000	2001	2002	2003	2004
Newfoundland	927	945	929	975	992
PEI	178	190	191	195	210
Nova Scotia	1,898	1,885	1,943	1,958	2,000
New Brunswick	1,153	1,179	1,185	1,224	1,262
Quebec	15,770	15,866	15,800	15,518	16,145
Ontario	21,176	21,482	21,735	21,738	22,067
Manitoba	2,082	2,093	2,077	2,063	2,078
Saskatchewan	1,567	1,549	1,564	1,526	1,529
Alberta	5,014	5,154	5,637	5,801	5,953
BC	7,943	8,105	8,243	8,348	8,257
Yukon	41	54	52	55	61
NW Territories	47	37	46	43	51
Nunavut	7	7	10	10	7
Total Canada	57,803	58,546	59,412	59,454	60,612

Source: Southam Medical Database, CIHI. Available at: http://secure.cihi.ca/cihiweb/en/ AR14_2002_tab3_e.html.

5.2   Nurses

There is a strong belief across Canada that there is a nursing crisis and yet there is less agreement on exactly what this means and various opinions on what to do about it. While a number of reports have been released that describe and analyze the issues, they have tended to reflect the perspectives of the sponsoring organization rather than being a national attempt to resolve workforce problems. The issues associated with the nursing workforce are particularly complex and dynamic and involve multiple stakeholders, including governments, employers, professional associations, unions, and educators.

The supply of nurses, their quality and competency, and their retention in jobs and in the profession are all dependent upon many different factors, including educational capacity, clinical training opportunities, entry-to-practice standards, support for new graduates, efficient deployment patterns, continuing education opportunities, and supportive work environments. In 1999 and 2000 a consultation paper for discussion by stakeholders, was developed by the Working Group on Nursing Resources and Unregulated Health Care Workers, a sub-committee of the Federal/Provincial/Territorial Advisory Committee on Health Human Resources (ACHHR). This initial document offered an analysis of various perceptions held by the different stakeholders in order to establish a common understanding of the complexity of the issues. In the interim, The Nursing Workforce Study was commissioned by the ACHHR.[99] This study included a survey of deployment patterns as well as nursing education and supply in 1990 and 1997.

The ACHHR issued its report, titled The Nursing Strategy for Canada, in October 2000, with eleven strategies for change. Stakeholders throughout the health care system recognized the need to increase and improve nurse workforce planning. Foreign recruitment was not among the advocated strategies, as local production was highly favoured. Yet not much has changed today. Rural/ urban distributions remain problematic. Decreases in the absolute numbers of RNs accompanied by the increase in the absolute numbers of Canadians have led to decreases in nurse to population ratios in both rural and urban areas of Canada. In 2000, the overall nurse to population ratio stood at 75.6 nurses per 10,000 population – down from 82.0 in 1992. However, nurse to population ratios in rural areas were much lower: 62.3 versus 78.0 for urban areas.[100]

Figure 7: Percentage Growth in the Number of RNs Employed in Nursing, Canada, 1980-2003

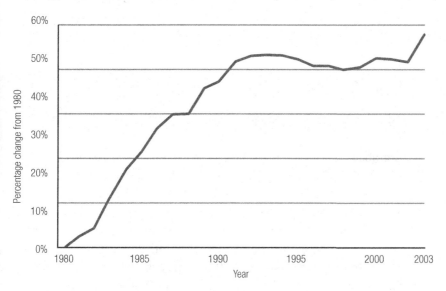

Source: CIHI, Workforce Trends of Registered Nurses in Canada, 2004, CIHI, Ottawa, 2005, p. 13.

While appreciable increases in nursing education across Canada have been implemented in the last decade, there have been concurrent changes in transforming all RN diploma programs to Baccalaureate degree training. This has resulted in a decrease, at least in the short term, in the number of graduates from RN programs and the number entering the workforce, further compounding the problem of an aging workforce.[101]

The hospital sector remains the largest nursing employment sector for RNs in all regions of Canada, despite many years of restructuring and downsizing of acute care institutions. About two thirds of Canadian RNs work in a hospital. The remainder work in long-term care, the community sector and other areas, such as in schools, physicians' offices and in government.

While organized recruitment efforts from outside Canada have taken place on occasion, these have been limited and usually by individual employers. Some respondents noted that most of the international graduates in nursing arrived in Canada on "coat-tails," with spouse/partner as the principal immigration applicant. If employment opportunities are generally favourable in the province of landing, the foreign-trained nurse would be likely to seek employment and thus be registered and counted in that province. If not, we experience another instance of "brain waste," although there is no data indicating the extent to which this may be occurring, apart from estimates of the large number of foreign-trained nurses who fail to complete their qualifications for Canadian registration.[102] Finally, while statistics indicate a declining percentage of foreign-trained RNs employed in Canada (total), absolute numbers rose in 2004.

6 Brain Drain from Canada to USA and Other Countries

Each year about one per cent of Canada's total supply of physicians leaves to work abroad. Over the last 33 years, the actual annual number of Canadian émigré physicians has fluctuated between 200 and 800. Save a brief period from 1991-1997, over half of those who left eventually returned to Canada.[103] Emigration trends show there was actually a noticeable drop in the number of physicians who moved abroad over the six-year period of 1998-2003. In the period 1998 to 2003 an average of 500 physicians per year left Canada to work abroad compared to the higher average of 690 physicians leaving from 1992-1997. On the other hand, the numbers returning in the same period

1992-2003 have been steady throughout the entire 12-year period, averaging 275 physicians a year. In 2003, the last year surveyed by the Canadian Medical Association, there was an even greater drop in numbers of physicians leaving Canada. In more recent years, specifically from 1998-2003, over half of the physicians who left Canada therefore returned.

Table 10: Canadian Physicians Moving and Returning from Abroad, 1992-2005			
	Physicians who moved	Physicians who returned	Net loss
1992	689	259	430
1993	635	278	357
1994	777	296	481
1995	660	250	410
1996	726	218	508
1997	658	227	431
1998	568	319	249
1999	584	340	244
2000	420	256	164
2001	609	334	275
2002	500	291	209
2003	320	240	80
2004	262	317	+55
2005	186	247	+61
Totals	7,594	3,872	3,722

Source: Available at: http://www.cma.ca/multimedia/CMA/Content_Images/Inside_cma/Statistics/

Numerous respondents expressed serious concern over the widely reported shortages in health care professionals the USA will experience and the effect it may have on Canada, since it is expected that the USA will target Canada to fill its shortages. The predictions of a doctor shortage represent an abrupt about-face for the medical profession. For the past quarter-century, the American Medical Association and other industry groups predicted a glut of physicians and, as Canada did in the 1990s, worked to limit the number of new doctors. In 1994, the Journal of the American Medical Association predicted a surplus of 165,000 doctors by 2000.[104] Forecasts have now changed dramatically, calling for 10,000 additional physicians to be trained each year, in addition to the current total of 25,000. If nothing is done, it is predicted there will be a shortage of 85,000-200,000 physicians by the year 2020.[105] Shortages in nurses in the USA will be even more acute. The US Human Resources and Services Administration predicts a shortage of 400,000 to 700,000 by the year 2020 – 20 per cent below RN workforce requirements.[106] Canada (along with the UK and Australia) is seen as a prime target for recruitment to fill these shortages because Canadian health professionals have no trouble becoming licensed there, require no upgrade training, speak the same language and are culturally similar to their American counterparts. Given the United States' post 9/11 security concerns, Canada is perceived as a country comprised of low-risk citizens, and therefore a safe country from which to recruit.

One respondent expressed concern at the American recruitment tactic of paying off student loans of new health care graduates in exchange for time-limited commitments, offering them the chance to be immediately debt-free. New medical graduates in Canada typically owe around $100,000 upon graduation. Federal student loans do not provide sufficient funds to cover the costs of medical training which forces medical students to resort to private lenders. While there are domestic programs offering incentives (e.g. payment of student loans if one commits to four years in a rural community, or programs within the military) these may seem less enticing than the American recruitment offers. Canada may have to look at revising some aspects of its student loan programs to address these American initiatives.

7 Costs and Benefits to Canada and Source Countries

7.1 Benefits to Canada

Respondents spoke of numerous benefits obtained by Canada from the flow of health professionals to the country. One respondent explained how "South African nurses have a wealth of experience and sometimes greater scope of practice because of the South African context. Moreover their competencies are roughly equivalent to Canadians as they have been educated under a similar system, so the gain is really fairly high in Canada's perspective. The fact that these nurses speak English is also a benefit."

Other respondents referred to Canada benefiting from gains in new knowledge and specialized experience. As one explained, "doctors trained exclusively in Canada may not be able to appreciate some of the diseases and psychological and psychosomatic issues associated with an East Asian frame of mind whereas a doctor trained in that region would." It is hard to assess the benefits brought by such knowledge.

A small number of respondents further pointed out those newly credentialed foreign-trained health care professionals typically take positions in rural or difficult-to-fill regions of Canada and are therefore filling an important gap in Canada's health care system.

In financial terms, Canada almost certainly benefits substantially each time a foreign-trained physician or nurse immigrates to work in the Canadian health care system as each represents one less Canadian-trained health care professional funded by Canada. Although there is no hard data, the costs of training a Canadian nurse or physician through the entirety of their studies is almost certainly greater than the costs Canada incurs in examining, evaluating, offering additional practical and language training to, or licensing foreign-trained health care professionals. A small number of respondents felt the costs to Canada may well balance out but the overwhelming majority of respondents felt that Canada experienced a notable net gain each time a foreign-trained health care professional joined the Canadian health force.

7.2   Costs to Canada

Costs to Canada from the flow of health professionals to the country acknowledged by respondents largely involve the processes required to retrain and re-credential health care providers from developing countries:

- assessment of existing credentials and identification of training they would still need to be on par with Canadian trained health care professionals. This matter is of considerable concern to many interviewees (particularly credentialing of those who come of own accord, i.e. not recruited);

- retraining individuals (skills enhancement) paid by Canada;

- post-graduate training/residency; and

- language training.

One respondent gave an example of the costs of administering these programs in one Canadian province alone. In 2004-2005, this province committed $26 million towards its international medical graduate program. The program ensured that there were no costs borne by the individuals as they pursued post-graduate training and, in fact, the individuals earned the same salary as residents who were Canadian medical graduates. For those who required assessments only, the provincial government also paid a stipend during the assessment period. Individuals were therefore required to pay only medical council examination fees and for other exams they might have been required to take as a normal part of registration in the province. These costs were estimated by the respondent as "small in comparison to the cost that the province is paying on their behalf in order to assist them to become part of the system."

Foreign-trained physicians may enter practice without any Canadian post-graduate training or may spend a certain period of time in a post-graduate training or residency program. CIHI figures demonstrate that the number of foreign-trained physicians requiring residency or post-graduate training in Canada peaked in 1982 (with approximately 220 individuals) and decreased considerably by 2000 (with approximately 35 individuals).[107] This indicates that greater numbers of foreign-trained physicians have sufficient training when arriving to Canada and can begin work upon licensing. This logically means that Canada now has fewer costs associated with training foreign-trained physicians.

In connection with this last point, one respondent roughly differentiated the costs to Canada according to three different categories of foreign-trained physicians. The first category can be integrated without any costs at all because they are highly trained and receive immediate licensing. These represent a net savings to Canada ranging from $950,000 (for a family physician) to $1.5 million (for a specialist), based on 1994 estimates of the full infrastructure costs associated with medical training (faculty and staff salaries, physical facilities, laboratories and so on.)[108] The second category requires six to twelve months of residency training to come to par with Canadian standards. A residency is estimated to cost approximately $50,000 - $70,000. The third category consists of individuals unable to practice without going through extra training, exams and residencies. It is estimated that there are 3,000 - 4,000 individuals falling within this category in the province of Ontario alone. The absence of funding for training and shortages in residencies results in "brain waste."

Numerous respondents raised the matter of a frustrating brain waste phenomenon where foreign-trained health care professionals are not able, or do not seek, to pass exams and gain credentials to practice in Canada. While no study has been undertaken on the profiles of individuals falling into this category, respondents spoke anecdotally of capable foreign-trained nurses and other health practitioners working in unskilled or unrelated jobs. It was suggested that Canada should at least seek to maximize the potential of these foreign-trained health care professionals who clearly decided to leave their countries and yet are not working in their area of training in Canada, despite shortages in this market.

Numerous respondents also took the opportunity to point out that Canada suffers from its own brain drain, with highly-subsidized, Canadian-trained health care professionals emigrating to other countries. Included in this exodus are foreign-trained health care professionals who have obtained training and credentials through brief emigration to Canada. Some respondents remarked that such individuals actually cost Canada as investments that are made in training, evaluating and/or credentialing are short-lived. Using the snapshot of the year 2003, we see that just under a third of physicians moving abroad from Canada were foreign-trained, indicating Canada is a temporary stop for a considerable number.[109]

Table 11: Emigration and Re-Entry of Physicians in Canada, 2003	
Total number of physicians in Canada who moved abroad	320
Number who graduated from Canadian medical schools	212
Number who graduated from foreign medical schools	95
Total number of physicians who returned from abroad	240
Number who graduated from Canadian medical schools	198
Number who graduated from foreign medical schools	40
Source: Summarized from Tables 14.0, 15.0, 17.0 and 18.0 in CIHI, Supply, Distribution and Migration of Canadian Physicians 2003, CIHI, Ottawa 2004.	

7.3 Costs to Source Countries

The costs to SSA source countries of brain drain have been acknowledged in numerous reports and are the reason why the WHO and World Bank have called for urgent action to reduce the phenomenon, and why nations such as the UK, Canada and others are adopting measures to the same end. Losses can be counted in terms of:

• government investment in training health professionals;

- health professionals to provide care;

- tutors to teach new students;

- increased burden on remaining health professionals; and

- diminished ability to provide health care.[110]

Respondents principally listed the direct costs of training health profession-als and loss of trained individuals to train new recruits (loss of teaching staff) as costs to source countries. The cost of training a doctor in South Africa, for example, has been estimated at $150,000 which translates into a major loss to the country.[111]

7.4   Benefits to Source Countries

The benefits to source countries most frequently cited are remittances by for-eign-trained health care professionals to their families, and investments in their home markets. In a recent UK survey, more than half of the foreign-trained nurses in that country reported that they regularly send money to their home country. In many cases this regular remittance amounts to a significant propor-tion of their total income: half of the nurses from South Africa participating in the survey reported they were sending a quarter or more of their monthly income back home.[112]

Numerous respondents in this study, including the sample of foreign-trained physicians in Canada, referred to significant remittances made to families back home. Remittances were largely to support family members and to pay off investments in their home countries (principally the family home). Remittances therefore typically represent private welfare gains and do very little to offset the public health investment losses incurred by source countries upon the emigra-tion of health care professionals.[113] A British report similarly notes with respect to health professionals who have migrated internationally that there is little evi-dence to suggest that the private positive benefit accrued by families through remittances by skilled health workers compensates in any way for the loss of capacity to the health system.[114] While the WHO suggests devising a system in which remittances could be channelled directly into the health system as a form of compensation,[115] this would likely be riddled with difficulties, not the least of which would be to account for remittances since large amounts move through informal channels.[116] Strong incentives schemes would also have to be devised to convince individuals to remit to the State rather than directly to their families.[117]

By contrast, another UK report on Ghanaian health care professionals in the UK found that many migrants remit funds with the express plan to return and finally settle back in Ghana. The conclusion of the authors of the report is that allowing health workers to remit and invest in the country of origin is "likely to be effective in reversing the spiral of migration."[118] This may depend, however, on the extent to which immigrant health professionals establish themselves in the receiving country, which can also depend on their age and family status.

7.5 Estimating Canada's Financial Obligation for HHR Investment in Africa: A Discussion

Canadian respondents almost universally rejected the concept of reparation for the costs to source countries, of foreign-trained health professionals. Nonetheless, the issue of reparation remains a policy option of considerable interest to African countries. It is also a policy option proposed and encouraged by the WHO.[119] There is thus a need for a brief discussion of differing arguments for how such reparations might be considered or calculated, in the context of reducing "push factors" from SSA countries by strengthening health systems.

There are two perspectives regarding Canada's involvement in strengthening African health systems: first, strong health systems are an integral part of achieving the Millennium Development Goals (MDGs) and Canada's own targets for official development assistance (ODA); facilitating the human right to health; and successfully addressing the growing burden of disease in Africa. In other words, Canada's obligation is rooted in its pre-existing initiatives and agreements, regardless of the additional problem of health human resource migration from Africa to Canada. Two general comments are necessary: first, any additional finances disbursed to African source countries to compensate for their loss of health human resources would likely flow through the ODA envelope; second, Canada, despite repeated pledges to provide at least 0.7 per cent of its gross domestic product to foreign aid, has consistently failed to do so and is one of the few remaining donor countries that has not committed itself to meeting this target by a certain date.[120]

The second perspective is that Canada is obligated to intervene due to the significant number of health workers who have migrated from Africa to Canada. While not all of these individuals migrated due to active recruitment, the line between active and passive recruitment is very thin. Regardless of the reason for the out-migration of these personnel, the result has been of significant benefit to Canada and a significant detriment to the health systems and people left behind. There are two possibilities for a reasonable determination of Canada's contribution on this basis: a calculation based upon the amount of out-migration, and a calculation based upon the health impact of that out-migration. Both would have to be assessed on a national basis, but linked to a broader regional perspective.

The first proposal is relatively straightforward. Let us say that South Africa calculates that it requires two billion dollars to replace the health workers who have left the country. If Canada has received twenty percent of these emigrating health workers then its share of the burden is twenty percent. Extending this discussion to the regional level, let us say that Canada has received thirty percent of Sub-Saharan Africa's health workers. Canada would be responsible for thirty percent of the cost of regional HHR initiatives, such as regional migration monitoring facilities, regional HHR planning initiatives, or the creation of regional institutions to address these issues. This appropriately links compensation on a nation-by-nation basis to that of the overall needs of the region.

The second proposal is more complicated and more controversial. It retains the focus upon a nation-by-nation assessment of Canada's obligation, but also weights the relative importance of the resource lost. Some nations need their health workers more than others and some health workers are worth more than others. For example, the loss of a physician who is involved with the training of other physicians arguably may be greater than the loss of one who is not, as the long-term impact of losing individuals who build capacity will be very significant. In Africa, as in Canada, rural physicians are harder to retain, and therefore may be worth more to that nation than urban physicians. (Although the loss of an urban physician may then become an in-country "pull" for urban migration by a rural physician.) As well, some nations may have a more difficult time replacing their lost workforce than other nations, due to the makeup of their populations or structure of their education system. Therefore, not only are some physicians more valuable than others, but some nations need their physicians less than others. This is not to say that physicians are unimportant, but rather that the health impact of the loss of a physician from one country may be greater than if that physician was recruited from another. This calculation requires a weighted valuation of the physicians from a specific nation. For example, if it costs less for South Africa to train a replacement physician and it is better able to deal with the loss of physicians than other countries, there is less impact upon the South African medical system and it requires less compensation for the loss of its physicians. Nations where the impact is greater deserve greater compensation.

Determining impact is difficult. It is unlikely that the data exists for this proposal to be implemented, but it is the fairest proposal. If a set amount of compensation per physician was to be determined it would have to adjust, inter alia, for the following factors: involvement in training other medical professionals, amount of experience, rural or urban experience, the specific discipline and its relative importance within the given nation, the ability of the nation to replace the individual and the expected remaining years of service.

The preceding argument requires the determination of a base compensation for each physician. This can be calculated in two ways. It can either be based upon the cost of training the replacement physician within that system, or it can be linked to the net financial benefit to the recipient country. The cost of training would vary from nation to nation and type of practice. Estimates by informed individuals suggests a figure in the $60,000 - $150,000 range to train a physician in Africa. The costs of training physicians within Canada are significantly more expensive, ranging (in 1994 $) between $950,000 and $1.5 million.[121] The other piece of the puzzle is to calculate exactly how much it costs to bring an internationally trained physician up to the standard of the Canadian medical system. The net benefit to Canada, for every foreign physician who migrates to Canada, is the cost of training a comparable Canadian minus the cost of upgrading that physician's skills. For example, if it requires $150,000 to train to Canadian licensure standards a South African family physician the net benefit to Canada is $950,000 - $150,000 = $800,000. A reasonable amount of compensation might lie somewhere between Canada's net benefit and the cost of training a physician within the migrant's country of origin.

In conclusion, any equitable compensation should be linked to the number of health workers who have emigrated from the source to the recipient nations. A nation-by-nation analysis would further ensure that any compensation arrangement agreed upon would recognize the diverse nature and health needs of African nations.

8 Policy Options

There is little disagreement about the nature of the "crises" in global health human resources, exacerbated by the flow of HHRs from developing to developed countries. But there is little agreement on what can be done to remedy it, in terms of what is politically feasible and who should assume responsibility.

8.1 Codes of Practice for Ethical Recruitment

None of the organizations interviewed had adopted a code of practice for ethical recruitment, although a small number had issued statements against the active recruitment of health care professionals from developing countries with acute shortages of health care practitioners. Indeed, very few concerned organizations had formally acknowledged the extent to which Canada depends on foreign-trained health care professionals to sustain the Canadian health care system or that it poses a problem to developing countries.

Mention of the Commonwealth Code of Practice for the International Recruitment of Health Workers was made by a few respondents. The Commonwealth set a precedent for action in 2003 when it agreed on guidelines for the international recruitment of health care professionals in a manner that takes into account the potential impact of such recruitment on services in source countries. Respondents cited the Commonwealth Code as a positive measure although they stressed its voluntary (non-binding) character. The Code provides guidelines for the international recruitment of health workers which, for example:

- discourage targeted recruitment;

- discourage recruitment of health care workers who have an outstanding obligation to their country;

- encourage the mutuality of benefits where receiving countries provide something in return (e.g. technical assistance, compensation, transfer of technology, financial assistance); and

- facilitate the return of recruits who wish to do so.

The Commonwealth Code also addresses the effects of international recruitment. Accordingly, it suggests:

- dialogue between developed and developing countries to balance needs of developed countries to recruit and developing countries to retain staff due to shortages;

- bilateral agreements to regulate the recruiting process; and

- that all employment agencies should be bound by this Code and that governments should set up regulatory systems for recruitment agencies and implement mechanisms to detect non-compliance.

In a recent WHO Bulletin, the Commonwealth Code of Practice was criticized for the fact that "it has been signed primarily by developing country members rather than importers of health workers such as Australia, Canada and the United Kingdom, who are reluctant to make a formal commitment to provide compensation or reparations."[122] In response to such criticisms, the Government of Canada has argued that its failure to sign is a result of its complex federation status effectively requiring approval by all provinces and territories; but that Canada and the provinces have expressed support for the Code and its principles which constitutes a de facto endorsement. The stakeholder organization most familiar with the Commonwealth Code nonetheless expressed concern over its uncertain impact to date. Other concerns about the Code include:

- the objective of protecting developing countries' health systems is overshadowed by its protection of employment rights of migrants;[123]

- systems for implementing the use of the instruments need to be strengthened; and

- no provision is made for a strategy for implementation nor a system for monitoring and evaluation.[124]

One informant made reference to the Melbourne Manifesto, a code of practice for the international recruitment of health care professionals adopted by delegates to the World Organization of National Colleges, Academies and Academic Associations of General Practitioners/Family Physicians (WONCA) meeting in Melbourne, Australia on 3 May 2002. The Manifesto acknowledges that the response of wealthier countries experiencing shortages in skilled health care professionals is too often to recruit from poorer countries rather than training sufficient numbers of their own. It recommends, inter alia, time-limited exchanges, where health professionals from developing countries come to practice and enhance skills in Canada and Canadians go to work in those countries and government support for medical training programs in developing countries. These recommendations align closely with the option of pursuing multilateral or bilateral agreements. They were also frequently mentioned by the foreign-trained physicians working in Canada, including support for job-sharing with someone in their source country, financial support from Canada for the first year or two if they returned to their source country to resume their practice there, and greater support and opportunity for short- and medium-term (two to six months or longer) periods of work back in their source country.

In comparative terms, the Melbourne Manifesto is much more specific in its guidelines and therefore more useful as a tool than the Commonwealth Code. However, judging by absence of reference, neither the Commonwealth Code nor the Melbourne Manifesto seemed to be known or considered seriously by most informants in this study. As such, these voluntary, multilateral agreements have failed to make any significant impact.

Yet when participants were asked whether they would support the adoption of a voluntary or mandatory code of practice, responses were generally positive. Respondents qualified that the codes should be voluntary, with the exception of one informant who indicated either approach would be acceptable. Some noted that voluntary codes, such as the one adopted in the UK, have not worked because of their voluntary nature. At the same time, they expressed concern that mandatory codes were unlikely to be ratified. A small number of respondents further noted that proper enforcement of such a code would require significant funding.

Newer principles, commonly referred to as the "London Declaration," were agreed upon at an international conference on the global health workforce organized on 14 April 2005 by the British Medical Association in association with the Commonwealth. Participants included the American Medical Association, the American Nurses Association, the Commonwealth Medical Association, the Commonwealth Nurses Federation, Health Canada, the Medical Council of Canada, the Royal College of Nursing and the South African Medical Association. The conference agreed on the following four key points:

- All countries must strive to attain self-sufficiency in their health care workforce without generating adverse consequences for other countries;

- Developed countries must assist developing countries to expand their capacity to train and retain physicians and nurses, to enable them to become self-sufficient;

- All countries must ensure that their health care workers are educated, funded and supported to meet the health care needs of their populations; and

- Action to combat the skills drain in this area must balance the right to health of populations and other individual human rights.

8.2   Improved Health Human Resources Planning in Canada

All organizations felt strongly that better health human resource planning in developed countries is a top priority and many further indicated that they were actively pursuing this aim. Respondents felt that better planning human resources to ensure an adequate stock of Canadian-trained health care professionals would be the best manner in which to reduce the inflow of foreign-trained health care professionals that is so damaging to developing countries.

The general consensus was that Canada should increase the number of training spots in schools of medicine and nursing. One respondent cited an average of five to nine applicants for every medical spot in Canada, resulting in wasted potential for self-sustainability or an ensured steady stock. Respondents complained that Canada is not doing a good job predicting and planning its resource needs. As one noted, "Every ten years we say we have too many and we close down enrolments and then every five years thereafter we say we have too few and open up enrolments again and there's never a proper fit."

Respondents felt that improved planning of human resources in health care would lead to increases in the stock of Canadian-trained physicians and nurses. This would necessarily lead to a decrease in the need for foreign-trained professionals. The conclusion to be derived is a fundamental and widespread understanding that, despite the absence of active recruitment, foreign health care professionals are aware of Canada's shortages and use the opportunity offered by shortages to emigrate. Once the need for foreign-trained professionals is reduced, it is believed that fewer will seek to leave their countries and jobs to emigrate to Canada. A strongly supported option to help SSA countries overcome the problem of brain drain is to improve self-sustainability. This option nonetheless requires a reduction in push factors in source countries, otherwise health care professionals will continue to leave for other countries even if Canada is no longer a strong "pull."

Most provinces have already reacted to the shortage by making substantial increases in medical and nursing school enrolments. However, the increases are not enough (especially in light of anticipated recruitment of Canadian health professionals by health systems in the USA facing a numerically much larger projected deficit), are financially costly and are difficult to sustain. The Canadian Medical Association, in collaboration with a number of other medical professional groups, is calling on Canadian governments to create a $1 billion "health human resources reinvestment fund" to ensure an adequate supply of domestically trained health care professionals. The president-elect of the CMA is critical that "we don't have a policy that Canada should be self-sustaining (...) we're poaching from other jurisdictions."[125]

Respondents suggested stepping up efforts to license foreign-trained health care professionals. The priority target group mentioned by a number of respondents and in various reports by provincial and national medical associations are non-nationals who have obtained their degree abroad, have immigrated to Canada but who have difficulty obtaining certification in Canada. Respondents encouraged the creation of mechanisms to assist these individuals to meet Canadian standards. The point was also made that it is not always medical upgrading that is required but language which must be enhanced.

Another group of similar concern consists of Canadians who have obtained their training outside of Canada. The College of Physicians & Surgeons of Ontario (CPSO) reports that, in Ontario alone, approximately 200 Ontarians graduate each year from medical schools outside of Canada. Roughly 100 Canadians are enrolled each year in four schools of medicine in Ireland alone.[126] Fifteen percent of the 1,929 medical doctors entering into their first year of residency in the 2004-2005 school year were Canadian citizens or permanent residents who obtained their MD training abroad.[127] These are the lucky ones able to obtain residencies. Calls were made by some respondents for improved mechanisms to evaluate degrees obtained by Canadians abroad and, in the event of inadequate equivalencies, to make residency and upgrading available so that they can meet Canadian standards. The CPSO has similarly issued recommendations urging the government to assess the qualifications of all foreign-trained medical graduates, significantly expand training opportunities and eliminate existing barriers.[128]

8.3   Multilateral and Bilateral Agreements

The New Partnership for Africa's Development (NEPAD) health strategy specifically refers to the necessity of developing some form of bi- or multilateral agreement to manage the brain drain of professionals from African countries. Agreements would entail measures for managed migration so that there would be no or little net loss to source countries.

Respondents were ambivalent towards this option, foreseeing numerous challenges. Most felt it would require a lot of organization and would give rise to many practical problems, the most evident being the monitoring of the agreements. As such agreements typically provide for the return of health professionals to the source country after two to three years abroad, others foresaw problems stemming from health professionals refusing to return once established with their families in Canada. This would appear to be valid concern given that foreign-trained health professionals tend to be older upon migration, and therefore more likely to have children. This was further corroborated by respondents who consistently described foreign-trained health care professionals coming to Canada as older and with young families.[129] This evidence also supports study findings that better educational opportunities for children in Canada present a significant pull factor for migration.

Others pointed out that less ethical countries could simply "free-ride" on any bilateral agreements. The existence of bilateral agreements would result in less competition from typical receiving countries which would otherwise take a number of health professionals from the pool.

Respondents felt that, if such agreements were to take place, they would more likely be in the form of Memoranda of Understanding (MoUs). While MoUs would be more difficult to enforce, the other option of drafting and adopting a framework convention would be particularly long in the making, complicated and with uncertain results.

One respondent stressed that multilateral agreements would be particularly complex and near-to-impossible to monitor and oversee, but that bilateral agreements could work with the right framework behind them. Some felt such agreements are not needed and that they would be a waste of time, effort and resources. One respondent flatly observed, "We live in a global market and professionals are free to move. It is up to the developing countries to set their own policies on how to deal with them." This sentiment, however, fails to account for Canada's health human resources planning errors creating a "pull," the role of immigration policy in easing entry for skilled professionals, and Canada's obligations under the right to health.

Some respondents made suggestions on the content of such agreements. Suggested provisions would:

- encourage the return of health workers to source countries, providing for a set period of service in Canada;

- secure the positions of persons coming for a set period of time to Canada so they would be easily re-employed upon their return;

- facilitate two-way staff flows – exchanges of health professionals between both countries, so that source countries would not experience a loss of staff and at the same time would benefit from new knowledge brought by Canadian health practitioners;

- foresee the payment of a penalty by either country breaking the terms of the agreement; and

- prevent poaching by a third party through the provision of a monetary penalty.

A small number of respondents remarked that it would be in Canada's best interests to support the regular conclusion of such agreements as a means to stem Canada's own brain drain of health care professionals to the USA and other countries, especially in light of the reported phenomenal shortages the USA will experience in the near future. Bilateral agreements might well protect Canada against losing any gains it is trying to make in balancing health human resources planning.

Following the example of the UK, the Canadian Government and a handful of health care regulating and monitoring bodies have begun to draft a memorandum of understanding between Canada and South Africa regarding the international recruitment of health care professionals. A Canadian "scoping mission" to South Africa to assess the possibility of such an MoU took place in November 2005.

8.4 Reparation Payments and Restitution to Source Countries

Respondents were asked for their views on the idea of financial reparation to source countries for training and health system losses from the migration of health professionals. Interview respondents voiced the greatest indication of rejection. Most respondents felt financial reparations would be "delicate," "difficult," and even "impossible" to oversee. Some clarified their opposition, explaining that, as there is no explicit public policy to recruit from these countries, Canadians would not want to reimburse for persons they had not "stolen" or "poached" in the first place. In their view, many foreign-trained health care workers were coming to Canada of their own initiative, having sought and been offered jobs prior to immigrating. They expressed concern that Canadians would feel that, since they decided to come to Canada on their own, there would be no reason why Canada should pay another country for their personal decision to migrate.

Ultimately, respondents believed public opinion matters and that, prior to any discussion on reimbursement, greater clarity was needed on how foreign health care providers come to Canada (Are they self-motivated? Or are they recruited?) and the real dollar costs involved in admitting foreign-trained health care providers, assessing their credentials, and retraining them where necessary.

The majority of respondents completely dismissed financial restitution as a viable option. Most made the point that the rotating door or circulation phenomenon – where countries, including Canada, lose health care providers through emigration and gain others through immigration – meant that foreign-trained practitioners in Canada could leave the country. Enough foreign-trained physicians in Canada emigrate to validate this concern. As foreign-trained health care workers were not bonded to Canada, they would be free to migrate to a third country, with Canada having paid their tab for reparations and subsidized their credentialing and re-training. Seeking repayment by the third party country would be even more difficult and placing foreign-trained practitioners on bonds upon arrival to Canada was frowned upon. Many respondents, while sensitive to the particular costs to source countries of the loss of skilled health care professionals, also argued that it was not reasonable or fair to single out the health care workers from the larger problem of the emigration of all types of skilled professionals from SSA countries. This logic would extend reparation for the loss of all skilled professionals who migrate from one country to another, creating a political, economic and accounting problem of such complexity as to be unimaginable in practice.

A UK report assessing policy options to reduce health professional migration also put forward the option of restitution equivalent to the salaried value of health workers employed in receiving countries.[130] Interestingly, the option was examined at a recent conference on health professional migration hosted by the BMA. All Commonwealth countries receiving migrants and the USA reportedly considered restitution a non-starter.[131]

8.5   Increased Training of Auxiliary Workers in Source Countries

Respondents were asked their views on another possible option: increasing training of auxiliary (lower-skilled) workers in source countries, thereby decreasing their attractiveness to health systems in receiving countries. Auxiliary workers would still be of enormous benefit to source countries with serious deficits in health care workers but these individuals would not likely gain entry into Canada on the merit of their training.

Views differed on this option, although the majority indicated strong opposition. Some believed it would result in a less trained medical force which could be more detrimental to the country's health care system. Others argued in a similar vein that the fragmentation of the health work force through the development of ad hoc groupings of sub-professional categories would be somewhat problematic as it would tend to result in the "de-skilling" of some professionals. One foreign-trained respondent found the idea verging on racist, arguing that while Western countries would likely continue receiving physicians and nurses from SSA countries (since this option would have no effect on reducing their migration), SSA source countries would be left with inferior health care workers to care for their populations.

Others judged it to be a good idea since there are typically not enough support health care workers in many source countries and that these could provide a great deal of basic treatment. As one respondent noted, "We focus on training the top end to the detriment of putting some of these lower end supports in place and I think it would be highly effective."

8.6 Restrictions on Health Professional Migration from Underserved Source Countries

Respondents were asked if their organizations would support restricting the migration of health professionals from SSA and other developing countries with severe deficits in health care workers. Restrictions could ostensibly be applied by placing health practitioners seeking to emigrate from underserved source countries on a low priority or points list.

All respondents were opposed to this solution. Respondents firmly believed in migration as an individual right which should not be discriminated by place of origin and profession. They followed up on this view with the argument that, as long as strong push factors in source countries existed, migration would continue. There would also always be a degree of "natural mobility" with health care professionals and others seeking to improve their quality of life.

8.7 Bonding of Health Care Professionals

The notion of bonding would require graduate health professionals to remain in service in their countries of training upon graduation as a way of repaying for the government-funded portion of their education. The bond would likely be for a number of years of service in a specific location, and may include a penalty if broken. This option could be applied to health care workers both in source countries and Canada. Respondents felt it was up to source countries to decide if bonding their health care workers would be a suitable and effective way to stem the drain of health care workers from their countries. While some said they would support such arrangements, it was made clear that this was beyond their mandate and ultimately not their business.

Bonding of new graduates in source countries would not conceivably be useful in stemming migration; health care professionals (at least physicians) are older when they migrate to Canada and would already have completed their period of bonding (Table 12). In the year 2003 only 5 per cent of newly graduated physicians practicing in Canada (less than five years since graduation) graduated abroad. As we know that somewhere between 20 and 30 percent of physicians in 2003 graduated abroad, we can deduce that foreign physicians do not typically migrate until later in their medical careers.

Table 12: Physicians by Year Since and Place of M.D. Graduation and Percent Distribution, Canada, 2003		
Years since MD Graduation	Place of graduation	
	Canada	Foreign
1 to 5	95%	5%
6 to 10	93%	7%
11 to 15	87%	13%
16 to 20	82%	18%
21 to 25	76%	24%
26 to 30	75%	25%
31 to 35	64%	36%
36 years and over	57%	43%
Source: Adapted from CIHI, Supply, Distribution and Migration of Canadian Physicians, 2003, CIHI, Ottawa, 2004.		

A UK study on the brain drain of health professionals examined and ultimately rejected bonding as a means of reducing migration. It reports that "[i]n circumstances where opportunities to move abroad are widely available, coercive measures taken in countries of origin to prevent departure appear to have been largely ineffective, and, unless they are widely accepted as legitimate, may increase pressures to leave."[132] Graduates prefer to pay the fines and break community service obligations. High inflation in source countries results in significant drops in the real cost of fines. For instance, in Ghana, where doctors are bonded to serve for five years or be in default to pay back training fees, the bond of 3,300 Ghanaian cedis worth 13 months' salary five years ago is now only worth five months. Moreover, many doctors leave without paying their bond since the policing of the bond is poor.[133]

Numerous respondents noted that bonding arrangements are already in effect in Canada. There was general consensus that such arrangements are worthwhile but that they should remain optional. Importantly, a buy-out clause must be available whereby a penalty could be paid if the bond (contract) terminated early. Others remarked that Canada should consider such bonds to minimize its own brain drain to the USA (or to the UK); several respondents also indicated they like would to see pan-Canadian policies in place to reduce inter-provincial brain drain.

8.8   Health System Strengthening in Source Countries

Health systems strengthening in SSA countries would result in far fewer push factors. This option was widely supported by respondents as a preferred measure to end brain drain. However, respondents also quickly noted that, for the most part, this option was largely out of their control and required policy action and involvement of donors and other multilateral institutions. On the other hand, some organizations cited examples of how they have already been involved through their networks in capacity building, skills training and policy instruction in developing countries and that they would continue to do so. Such efforts already take place. For instance, through the Association of Universities and Colleges of Canada (AUCC), the University of Calgary in Canada has partnered with the University of Ghana on a project aimed at increasing Ghana's capacity to educate and train the nurses required to meet priority needs in the health sector in a sustainable manner. Similarly, the University of Alberta has teamed with Makerere University to improve the quality of health care delivery in Uganda through better management and orientation of health care workers toward primary health care.

Others emphasized that such efforts should be focused bilaterally and that, even under such an arrangement, it would be complex to orchestrate or support exchanges. As in the case of bonding, numerous respondents expressed that efforts to strengthen health care systems in source countries were the principal concern of these countries and had little to do with the mandates of their own organizations. They nonetheless indicated this was a policy option that could be promoted to, and gain broad political support from, most members or constituents of their organizations. Moreover, increased aid from Canada to the health systems in SSA countries (including but not restricted to source countries) was seen as a more viable means of compensating source countries than reparations. Whether Canadian health development assistance to source countries exceeds estimates of Canada's gains or source countries' losses from health professional migration is still under empirical assessment.

8.9 Human Rights Issues Surrounding the Brain Drain and Policy Options

Human rights are commonly mentioned in describing the motivations of health care professionals to migrate to seek a better life as their migration is partly rooted in human rights abuses. However, the international migration of health care professionals also results in the failure of source countries to implement human rights, particularly the progressive realization of the full enjoyment of the right to health. In source countries critically lacking health human resources, the migration of such professionals has a catastrophic impact on their ability to provide adequate health care delivery, which is one of several core obligations under the right to health. SSA countries have considerable responsibility for some of this failure, including voluntary under-financing of public health systems, misuse or corrupt appropriation of public finances, "inverse care" distribution in which wealthier areas have a higher per capita proportion of public health services than do poorer ones, poor economic planning or policy choices leading to growing income inequalities and decreased future economic security. But some of this failure is also a result of the negative impacts of earlier periods of structural adjustment conditionalities attached to loans from the international financial institutions whose decisions are dominated by the very developed nations now benefiting from the emigration of health professionals from SSA countries.[134] In an increasingly integrated global economy, domestic policy decisions are not always freely chosen.

The development and implementation of policy responses to health professional brain drain may have varied impacts on the human rights of individuals. A human rights analysis of these options can assist in the selection of the most appropriate measures to address the brain drain. Judith Bueno de Mesquita and Matt Gordon, in their report for Medact, convincingly advance that "[a]pplying a human rights approach to addressing international health worker migration can help ensure the maximum possible benefit in human rights terms."[135] Their analysis, together with that of the UN Special Rapporteur on Health, Paul Hunt, significantly informs the next section.

8.10 Inadequately Protected Rights in Source Countries Leading to Migration

It is abundantly evident in the literature on migration in general and brain drain specifically, and from our own interviews, that health care professionals are leaving their countries in Sub-Saharan Africa because their fundamental rights to work, to an adequate standard of living and to security, as well as others, are not secured.

Article 23(1) of the Universal Declaration of Human Rights, adopted in 1948, declares that "[e]veryone has the right to work, to free choice of employment, to just and favourable conditions of work and to protection against unemployment." In the overwhelming majority of cases, health professionals seek to migrate because these basic rights are violated or are clearly at risk of being violated.

Article 25(1) of the Universal Declaration further recognizes that

> Everyone has the right to a standard of living adequate for the health and well-being of himself and of his family, including food, clothing, housing and medical care and necessary social services, and the right to security in the event of unemployment, sickness, disability, widowhood, old age or other lack of livelihood in circumstances beyond his control.

Without a doubt, health care professionals in SSA countries, if they are able to obtain work and if they are paid on a regular basis, are better able to support themselves and their families than individuals without skills. However, the struggle to sustain an adequate standard of living as defined in Article 25(1) is persistent and its outcome uncertain. Moreover, in many cases individuals cannot depend on an adequate social security system to support them in the event of unemployment, illness or retirement.

The International Covenant on Economic, Social and Cultural Rights, adopted in 1966, further specified what the right to work entails. Article

6 reiterates the individual's right to work and gain a living while Article 7 recognizes that individuals must be ensured just and favourable conditions which require:

- Remuneration which provides all workers, as a minimum with:

  i. Fair wages...;

  ii. A decent living for themselves and their families;

- Safe and healthy working conditions;

- Equal opportunity... to be promoted; and

- Rest, leisure and reasonable limitation of working hours and periodic holidays with pay....

There are numerous international labour conventions also prescribing minimum conditions of work. For instance, the Forty-Hour Week Convention (Convention No. 44), adopted in 1936, prescribes that individuals should not work more than 40 hours a week such that the standard of living is not reduced as a consequence. Convention No. 117 on Social Policy (Basic Aims and Standards) of 1962 also states that:

> [A]ll possible steps should be taken by appropriate international, regional and national measures to promote improvement in such fields as public health, housing, nutrition, education... conditions of employment, the remuneration of wage earners... social security, [and] standards of public services....[136]

From our research into the push factors leading health professionals to migrate or consider migrating, the absence of respect for these conditions were repeatedly leading causes for departure. Failure to ensure respect for these minimum conditions constitute violations by SSA states of human rights norms.

Compounding this struggle to obtain an adequate standard of living and just and favourable working conditions is the threat to personal security that individuals face in many SSA countries. Both the Universal Declaration of Human Rights and the International Covenant on Civil and Political Rights stipulate that States must ensure that everyone has the right to security of person, recognizing the absence of security as an obstacle to the enjoyment of many other rights.

There is a clear and strong belief issuing from the stakeholder interviews and the abundant literature being produced on the brain drain of health care professionals that the cycle of movement from underdeveloped to developed countries will only begin to diminish when the root causes of migration are addressed. The Cairo Declaration and Programme of Action, adopted at the International Conference on Population and Development held in 1994, describes the complexity at hand, stating that "[t]he long-term manageability of international migration hinges on making the option to remain in one's country a viable one for all people."[137] It also recognizes that, to make this option viable, "countries of origin and countries of destination must cooperate."[138]

8.11 The Rights of the Professional to Leave and Enter a Country

Article 13(2) of the Universal Declaration on human rights is crystal clear with regards to an individual's entitlement to leave his/her country. The article provides that "[e]veryone has the right to leave any country, including his own, and to return to his country." Article 12(2) of the International Covenant on Civil and Political Rights of 1966 reiterates this right. However, paragraph 3 of this Article further provides that the above-mentioned right:

> [S]hall not be subject to any restrictions except those which are provided by law, are necessary to protect national security, public order, public health [emphasis added] or morals or the rights and freedoms of other, and are consistent with the other rights recognized in the present Covenant.

States are aware that these restrictions are to be applied only in dire situations. It is interesting, however, that no SSA or other country suffering from severe shortages in health care professionals owing to migration has attempted to restrict the right to leave on the grounds of protecting public health. If a country was to do so, the burden would be on it to prove the necessity for such severe action. An example of legitimate grounds for such a restriction on the rights to freedom of movement and to leave would be to contain highly infectious diseases. However, it is unlikely that restricting freedom of movement of health workers as a response to the brain drain would qualify as permissible grounds for limitation. Other States would likely condemn such limitation if other measures which did not restrict the enjoyment of human rights were not first adopted. The argument could easily be made, for instance, that the State's own domestic policies and malappropriation of resources contributed to the need to migrate and that these should be the first, less intrusive, measures to pursue.

Some SSA countries place bonds on health care and other types of professionals in attempt to restrict their movements. The bonds are an attempt to preserve a country's human resources and its investment in the education of these individuals. No bonding contract refuses health care professionals the right to leave their country, which would be contrary to international human rights law. Rather, departure necessarily leads to a rupture of the bond contract and individuals must pay a penalty for breaking it. The provision and enforcement of such a penalty is not a violation of human rights. In any case, developing countries typically find it hard to enforce the penalties.

In contradistinction to an individual's human right to leave any country, international human rights law does not provide for a "right to enter any country." Who is allowed to enter into a country and for how long is the absolute prerogative of the State according to the fundamental principle of international law on territorial sovereignty.[139] The conditions of entry into a country are reflected in its immigration policy which may change with governments and over time.

Canada has adopted a policy which fosters immigration. Canada's policy is highly favourable towards skilled individuals. As a result, it effectively discriminates (i.e. distinguishes or differentiates) on the basis of education and profession. However, the policy is not discriminatory on the basis of race, colour, sex, religion, political or other opinion, or national or social origin – grounds on which a State would be in violation if it discriminated for whatever reason with respect to individuals within its territory. Indeed, individuals requesting entry into Canada are not within Canada's jurisdiction and so these standards of discrimination do not even apply. However, the comparison demonstrates that, even if one argued these standards applied in immigration policies, Canada's policy would not be in violation of international human rights law. In conclusion, it cannot be said that Canada's immigration policy discriminating in favour of skilled professionals violates international law.

8.12 The Right to Health in Source and Recipient Countries

The human right to health is embodied in a variety of international declarations, covenants and plans of action. Most notably, Article 12 of the International Covenant on Economic, Social and Cultural Rights (ICESCR) proclaims "the right of everyone to the enjoyment of the highest attainable standard of physical and mental health," and specifically obligates States Parties (which is the term referring to countries bound by the Covenant) to ensure:

> [P]rovision for the reduction of the stillbirth-rate and of infant mortality and for the healthy development of the child; the improvement of all aspects of environmental and industrial hygiene; the prevention, treatment and control of epidemic, endemic, occupational and other diseases; and the creation of conditions which would assure to all medical service and medical attention in the event of sickness.

One hundred and fifty countries are States Parties to the Covenant, including Canada. Although state obligations are limited to the "progressive realization" of this right in view of available resources, all states must show measurable progress towards its full realization. In 2000 the Committee on Economic, Social and Cultural Rights issued General Comment 14 on Article 12, which both clarified the scope of the right and identified State obligations under it.

General Comment 14 sets out in paragraph 12 two frameworks with which to evaluate realization of the right to health. The first is constituted by the essential elements of the right, namely:

1. Availability (functioning public health and sufficient health care facilities, goods and services),

2. Accessibility (including non-discrimination and affordability),

3. Acceptability (respectful of human right to dignity and of confidentiality),

4. Quality (scientific/medical appropriateness, adequate personnel and training).

The state must ensure that an adequate number of health professionals are available in the country, are accessible to all, including those living in rural areas, and deliver health services of good quality in a culturally acceptable manner.

Canada accepts and licences foreign-trained health professionals because there is a significant shortage of domestically produced professionals and considerable under-served (rural) areas. Foreign-trained health professionals fill important gaps and, as a consequence, health care is made more available and accessible to Canadians. Canada is thereby better able to fulfill its obligations under the right to health in accepting foreign-trained health care professionals. In the case of developing countries, however, migration has the exact opposite impact on the State's ability to secure the right to health. The loss of health professionals through migration means that countries are unable to ensure availability, accessibility and quality. The emigration of health care professionals therefore contributes to their abrogation of obligations under the right to health.

8.13 Human Rights Obligations of Recipient Countries

The second framework of General Comment 14 regarding health is provided by states' obligations.[140] Internationally, States Parties to the ICESCR must respect the right to health in other countries, for instance by refraining from using sanctions or embargoes to restrict the flow of adequate medicines and medical equipment to countries in need. This obligation also implies that when concluding other international agreements, States Parties "should take steps to ensure that these instruments do not adversely impact upon the right to health."[141]

As Paul Hunt, the UN Special Rapporteur on the Right to the Highest Attainable Standard of Health, explains in a recent report to the Commission on Human Rights, developed countries must respect the right to health in developing countries, specifying that at a minimum:

> [D]eveloped countries should ensure that their human resource policies do not jeopardize the right to health in developing countries. If a developed country actively recruits health professionals from a developing country that is suffering from a shortage of health professionals in such a manner that the recruitment reduces the developing country's capacity to fulfill the right to health obligations it owes its citizens, the developed country is prima facie in breach of its human rights responsibility of international assistance and cooperation in the context of the right to health.[142]

We have already explained that the distinction between active and passive recruitment is now blurred and that immigration programs and policies adopted by the Canadian Government make it easier for foreign-trained health professionals to come to work in Canada. Moreover, RHAs and clinics are actively recruiting in SSA countries in the traditional sense that they have targeted job announcements to health professionals in SSA countries through journals consulted by health professionals in the region.

States Parties to the ICESCR are also obliged to protect against infringements of this right by third parties such as corporations, by ensuring that third parties over whom they have legal or political influence respect the enjoyment of this right in other countries.[143] The obligation to fulfill requires the international community to support the progressive realization of this right through international assistance and cooperation.[144] ODA is one indicator of commitment to this obligation, although not the only one. With respect to the brain drain problem of SSA countries, Canada's failure to be self-reliant in domestic health human resources – creating a de facto "pull" on health care professionals from these countries that undermines their ability to progressively realize this right – arguably abrogates Canada's obligations under Article 12. This introduces an interesting legal and moral argument in support of reparations or, at a minimum, support to source countries that exceeds both their net losses benefits and Canada's net benefits arising from health care professional migration.

Hunt explains that, while the parameters of obligations of international assistance and cooperation are not completely clear in international law, it is incumbent on developed (and particularly recipient) States to help facilitate the enjoyment of the right to health in developing countries. Facilitation may be in the form of cooperation, support, aid, debt relief or other forms.

While individuals have the right to seek migration, the flow of health professionals from developing to developed countries – to the extent it results from the "push" and "pull" factors itemized earlier – is "inconsistent with developed countries' human rights responsibility of international assistance and cooperation, as well as other international commitments, including the Millennium Declaration and Goal 8."[145]

Bueno de Mesquita and Gordon recommend a human rights framework applicable to both source and recipient countries:

> Governments of countries of origin should improve rights in work for employees in their home country by strengthening their public systems, including better human resources planning. They should allocate a health share of the State budget commensurate with generally recognized international benchmarks and international agreements that they have signed up to. They should possibly adopt a range of other appropriate measures for meeting the right to health that are fast to implement in the short term, including auxiliary worker training, managed migration and a contract with health staff trained in the public system that invokes an obligation to the public health system for a period of time after training is completed. [Recipient] country governments should increase the resources available for countries of origin to strengthen health systems through positive and explicit acknowledgement of the

human rights impacts of hiring of international staff, known as restitution.[146]

Hunt, drawing his recommendations largely from the Plan of Action to prevent Brain Drain issued by Physicians for Human Rights, also advocates compensation, stating that, "depending on resource availability, States should provide aid to developing countries so as to facilitate access to essential health facilities, goods and services... Aid policies should include support for human resources in the health sector."[147] At the same time, he points out that it is fundamentally disingenuous to provide overseas development assistance, debt relief and other forms of aid with one hand while simultaneously taking health professionals trained at the expense of developing countries with the other.[148] Recipient and other developed countries must therefore address their own inadequate production and retention of health professionals, adhere to ethical recruitment principles, help strengthen health systems in source countries and promote macro-economic policies consistent with human rights."[149] Hunt also argues that such compensation would be just and that, with genuine political commitment, the difficulties in formulating this compensation and where it would go would not be insurmountable.[150]

He further suggests that, consistent with their responsibility of international assistance and cooperation, developed States should not apply undue pressure on developing countries to make GATS mode 4 commitments that are inconsistent with developing countries' obligations arising from the right to health. Hunt suggests a revision to mode 4 commitments so as to ensure that it will not have a negative impact on the right to health for all.[151]

In conclusion, the most appropriate response to the problems arising from migration of health care professionals is an integrated one, combining prevention (reducing the mitigating factors leading to migration) and ensuring that any improvements in the right to health are achieved without any negative repercussions to the right to health of others in source countries and without express limitation of any other rights, including freedom of movement and rights in work.

9 Measures Adopted by Other Countries

9.1 Australia

A recent report published by the Australian Health Ministers' Advisory Council (AHMAC) emphasized Australia's continuing dependence on foreign-trained doctors. The number of temporary resident foreign-trained doctors arriving in Australia to work in "areas of need," such as rural and remote areas, has increased over the last decade, from 667 in 1992 to 2,899 in 2001. Between four and five thousand foreign-trained nurses enter Australia annually. While many of these come from other wealthy countries, such as the United Kingdom, New Zealand, Canada, Ireland and Norway, source countries in the developing world, such as the Philippines, South Africa and Zimbabwe, are also important.[152]

Australia's reliance upon foreign-trained doctors is unlikely to diminish in the foreseeable future. This situation reflects past decisions of politicians and their advisers, health service administrators, those responsible for the provision of medical education programs and, by no means least, expectations and aspirations within the current medical workforce. Announcing Medicare Plus on 19 November 2003, the Federal Government promised to increase the number of available doctors, in part by recruiting appropriately trained overseas doctors.[153]

The biggest change in Australian immigration in the last decade is that, whereas it emphasized settlement migration in the five post-war decades, there has been a reversal with a number of new visa categories designed to attract temporary residents to work in the country. As a result there has been an exponential increase in non-permanent migration. Temporary migration is even more selective of skilled individuals than permanent migration. In mid-2004, there were nearly 600,000 people in Australia on a temporary status. Over half were skilled migrants and had the right to work. The temporary migration status is reportedly increasingly seen by both migrants and government as a prelude to permanent settlement in Australia. The overwhelming majority of migrants accorded permanent status in Australia remain in the country.[154]

Two hundred and eighty physicians from the SSA region gained permanent immigration status in Australia between 1993 and 2004. Of these, only 17 departed. 1,232 physicians from the SSA region were given temporary status in the same period and over half remain. The figures for nurses are even larger. Seven hundred and twenty one nurses from the SSA region were accorded permanent immigration status. All but 67 have remained in the country. 1,353 SSA nurses were accorded temporary status of which 805 have remained.[155]

9.2 Norway

Norway has an annual restriction on the number of nurses that can be recruited by its government agency, and this recruitment is based on government-to-government agreements. This approach of setting a state recruitment target has been shown to be effective in limiting the impact on source countries.[156]

9.3 The Netherlands

The Ghana-Netherlands Health Care Project has been cited as an example of a bilateral success story. Its objectives are to transfer knowledge, skills and experiences through short-term assignments and projects and practical internships for Ghanaians and to develop a centre for the maintenance of medical equipment in Ghana. It is meant to allow Ghanaian health professionals to offer services, conduct research and implement projects within Ghana.[157]

9.4 The United Kingdom

Reliance on overseas health practitioners is particularly apparent in the UK. Compared to other importer countries such as the USA, Norway, Ireland and Australia, the UK appears to be relatively more active in recruiting from developing countries.[158]

A survey of the Royal College of Nursing found that 13 per cent of nurses working in London alone are foreign-trained.[159] The majority of these come from the Philippines, Australasia, India, Ghana and Nigeria.[160] Another study adds South Africa, Zambia and Zimbabwe among the list of main source countries for nurses in the UK. Although noting a reduction in registrants from the Philippines and South Africa in recent years, it also acknowledges a continued increase from several other SSA countries.[161]

One in five doctors with full registration in the UK were trained in a developing country. Significant numbers come from South Africa, Pakistan, Egypt and Sri Lanka.[162] A report issued by the UK's Department for International Development (DFID) in 2004 cites a significant upward growth in inflow of doctors to the UK from developing countries in recent years.[163]

The Department of Health has introduced an ethical recruitment policy for National Health Service (NHS) employers. According to the UK, it was the first nation to produce international recruitment guidelines based on ethical principles and the first nation to develop a code of practice for international recruitment. The Code of Practice for the International Recruitment of Health Care Professionals, commonly referred to its abbreviated form as the NHS Code of Practice, stipulates that NHS trusts should not actively recruit from developing countries unless there is agreement with the government of the country. The Code lists the countries from which health care professionals should not be recruited, which comprises all developing countries, including South Africa. At the same time, there is also a Memorandum of Understanding between the UK and South Africa for the ethical recruitment of health care professionals.

The United Kingdom is widely regarded as setting the standards for bilateral agreements on ethical recruitment.[164] To date, such agreements exist with India, China, Pakistan and the Philippines. The agreements are largely target group-specific. For instance, the MOU between the UK and the Philippines pertains specifically to nursing.

9.4.1 NHS Code of Practice

The NHS Code of Practice was adopted by the UK's Department of Health in 2001. Its principal provisions are that it:

- applies to all health professionals;

- states that NHS employers are responsible for implementing the Code and managing the list of commercial agencies that adhere to the Code. Any recruitment agency that wishes to supply the NHS must comply with this Code;

- requires that developing countries not be targeted for recruitment;

- stipulates that active recruitment may only occur where bilateral agreements between countries exist; and

- restricts recruitment from over 150 developing countries. These countries must not be targeted for recruitment under any circumstances.

None of the organizations in the DFID case study on international recruitment reported actively recruiting from developing countries. However, the inflow of nurses from developing countries on the Department of Health list of countries proscribed for NHS active recruitment (e.g. Sub-Saharan Africa) continues to be significant.[165]

There are a number of passive recruitment forms which contribute to increasing numbers of international health workers going to the UK but which do not violate the NHS Code of Practice. A recent article on nursing in the UK found "[m]any nurses reporting that they initially worked in the UK for private sector employers (not regulated by the Code of Practice because the employers are not NHS) before moving quickly, sometimes immediately on completion of adaptation, to work in the NHS."[166] Another loophole occurs in that individuals who volunteer themselves by individual application may be considered for employment. This creates a grey zone as immigration policies may particularly facilitate or make way for immigration by these individuals who then need only present themselves to recruitment agencies. The DFID report also acknowledges the increased access to employment opportunities that has been created by the internet. Health workers in developing countries have become more aware of employment opportunities in developed countries because of access to recruitment agency and employer websites.[167]

The major limitation of the Code is that it does not cover the private sector, which continues to recruit from countries on the proscribed list. However, in December 2004, the UK Health Minister, John Hutton, announced that the UK would toughen the Code. The new Code entered into force at the end of 2005. It continues to prevent NHS hospitals from actively recruiting health care professionals from developing countries but extends the obligations to the private (independent) sector and to the employment of temporary and locum staff for the first time, thus closing a major loophole. The revised Code will mean the private sector will have to act more ethically. All independent sector companies providing NHS care will sign up to the Code of Practice through stipulations in their NHS contract. The Code also will be extended to cover 200 more recruitment agencies, to include agencies that supply domestic staff to the NHS.[168]

9.4.2   UK-South Africa Memo of Understanding

South Africa is among the countries listed in the NHS Code of Practice from which the UK cannot actively recruit health care workers. The Memo of Understanding, however, facilitates exchanges between the two countries.

Specifically, it provides that South African health care personnel can spend time-limited education and practice periods in organizations providing NHS services. Clinical staff from the UK work alongside health care personnel in South Africa, with particular emphasis on the rural areas. The Memo also provides for a bilateral twinning scheme between a South African and UK hospital. This has allowed 30 South African nurses to be placed in the UK for theoretical and practical training while senior nurses from the UK have worked in South Africa as mentors. A Canadian scoping mission to South Africa took place in November 2005 to determine the bases for, and value of, drafting a similar MOU between the two countries. Discussion between the two countries on this possibility is continuing.

10   Conclusions

Canada is heavily reliant on foreign-trained health care workers, with at least 22 per cent of physicians and 7 per cent of nurses in the country being foreign-trained. Some provinces are much more reliant on foreign-trained health professionals than others, with the less densely populated and highly rural prairie province of Saskatchewan having the highest percentage of foreign-trained physicians (over 50 per cent). Data reveals that Canada is less dependent on foreign-trained health professionals than most of its non-European OECD counterparts. However, it has a higher proportion of foreign-trained physicians from Sub-Saharan African countries, with South African physicians representing a large majority of these. It is therefore even more pressing and fitting that Canada consider its role in the brain drain of health professionals from Sub-Saharan Africa in particular, according special attention to South Africa.

Most Canadian respondents in this study felt that, in order to diminish the exodus of health professionals from the region, source countries have to tackle the factors pushing their health workers out. The recent announcement of South Africa's Health Minister that South Africa is committing to doing just that (e.g. by increasing pay and improving conditions of work) is a positive sign. The best means by which to reduce the drain, however, would be through concerted efforts from both sides – both Sub-Saharan African countries and Canada. A question this study has attempted to answer, is "how?" Attempts at answers were sought by asking key informants of stakeholder organizations closely involved in the Canadian health care system what policy options they would support as means to reduce the brain drain.

Respondents thought first and foremost of acting on the home front to reduce pull factors through improved health human resources planning. Severe short-ages of physicians and nurses in Canada would only continue to feed Canada's dependency on foreign-trained professionals, the lack of a clear deficit/inflow relationship notwithstanding. Stakeholder organizations would like to see increases in residencies and medical and nursing school enrolments as well as programs for re-training and licensing individuals having difficulty obtaining certification in Canada so that Canadians trained abroad and foreign-trained health professionals in Canada who are unable to practice can more readily join Canada's under-serviced health workforce. The Government of Canada, however, is taking steps to further facilitate the immigration of foreign-trained health care workers through the adoption of measures such as the Provincial Nominee Program and a new immigration points system favourable towards professionals such as physicians and nurses.

Respondents were supportive of, but less enthusiastic toward, the idea of Canada adopting voluntary or mandatory codes for the ethical recruitment of foreign-trained health care professionals. This largely stemmed from the belief held by most respondents that foreign-trained health professionals are not being actively recruited; rather, individuals are self-migrating. Gone are the days of Canadian-based recruitment agencies actively pursing foreign nationals to come to Canada. New arrivals are largely "recruited" by their own networks of colleagues already based in Canada, by individuals based in SSA countries with close ties to RHAs and hospitals, or through their own efforts, facilitated by the worldwide web and global journals. In this light, codes would be futile; and even if they were adopted they would prove difficult to monitor and enforce.

The unique structure of Canada's health care system makes it particu-larly difficult to determine where ultimate responsibility for the recruitment of health personnel lies and how it would be monitored. It is also the reason why it is difficult to obtain consensus on policy options to reduce reliance on foreign-trained health care workers. Respondents, however, were generally in consensus on the options they opposed. The idea of financial restitution to source countries for each of their health care workers Canada would obtain was the most widely rejected option. Respondents foresaw a plethora of com-plications in instituting such a measure. Respondents equally rejected the idea of placing restrictions on immigration to Canada for health care workers from underserved SSA countries. All believed such a measure would be a violation of fundamental human rights and contrary to Canadian values. The proposal to create bilateral or multilateral agreements between Canada and underserved SSA countries wherein conditions of migration would be strictly provided drew only very weak support. Respondents were primarily concerned with difficulties in overseeing the implementation of such agreements and the limitations they would place on the free movement and choice of individuals. The option of SSA countries placing bonds on their own health workers also gave rise to more concerns than support. Some respondents felt the bonds would be easily broken while others simply felt this was not a matter for Canadian stakeholders to comment on but for SSA countries to decide for themselves.

The final option presented to respondents was to strengthen health care systems in source countries. This option drew general support. However, while very few organizations were contributing to strengthening source country health care systems, or could even see how they could help, others simply felt this was a job for others and did not concern them.

It is clear that unless Canada and source countries take some action, the brain drain of health care professionals from Sub-Saharan Africa to Canada will continue. The greater fear is that, as Canada's shortages in physicians and nurses are exacerbated (as predicted), so will the brain drain. Unless measures are adopted, there is no indication or reason why trends in the sources of the drain to Canada will change; Canada will continue to receive significant numbers of health care professionals from Sub-Saharan Africa, a region itself so desperate for their skills.

So how will change occur? The survey of organizations with a stake in Canada's health care system demonstrated little support for many of the feasible options presented to them, seeming to find the negatives (impracticalities) of the options rather than the positives. They also repeatedly demonstrated the sentiment that the solutions were beyond their control and scope of influence, and lay with – for example – Canada's foreign or immigration policies. In reality any plausible chance for change likely lies in all these stakeholders playing their own respective roles in reducing the brain drain, and encouraging a broader intersectoral or "whole of government" approach to removing "push" and reducing "pull" factors. But our own conclusion is that they will have to be prompted and supported in doing so along the way.

Endnotes

1   World Bank Development Indicator. Available at: http://www.worldbank.org/htnl/schools/regions/ssa.htm.

2   WHO, Estimates of Health Personnel by Country. Available at: http://www.who.int

3   J. Bueno de Mesquita and M. Gordon, *The International Migration of Health Workers: A Human Rights Analysis* (London: Medact, 2004).

4   D. Dovlo, "Wastage in the Health Workforce: Some Perspectives from African countries" *Human Resources for Health* 3(6). Available at: http://www.human-resources-health.com/content/3/1/6.

5   Ibid.

6   See generally, e.g., D. Dovlo, "Migration and the Health System: Influences on Reaching the MDGs in Africa (and Other LDCs)" in *International Migration and the Millennium Development Goals* (New York: UNFPA, 2005), pp. 67-79.

7   Joint Learning Initiative, *Human Resources for Health: Overcoming the Crisis* (Cambridge: Global Health Trust, 2004).

8   See C. Ozden and M. Schiff, (eds.), *International Migration, Remittances and the Brain Drain* (New York: World Bank, 2006).

9   As examples of variations, in one of its briefs, the Centre for Global Development advances that increasing skill-focus of immigration policy in a number of leading industrialized countries is the leading cause for the migration of skilled professionals, Dovlo argues it is due to the demand for health workers in developed countries, and the World Bank attributes greater weight to push factors in underdeveloped countries leading skilled professionals to capitals of wealth. See D. Kapur and J. McHale, *The Global Migration of Talent: What Does it Mean for Developing Countries?* (Washington D.C.: Centre for Global Development, 2005); Dovlo, *op. cit.*, p. 67; and, J. Mora and J.E. Taylor, "Determinants of Migration, Destination, and Sector Choice" in C. Ozden and M. Schiff (eds.), *International Migration, Remittances, and the Brain Drain* (Washington World Bank, 2006), pp. 21-51.

10   See Ozden and Schiff, *International Migration, Remittances, and the Brain Drain.*

11   Reported in the presentation by Simi Arora of the IOM's Office of the Director of Health Human Resources at the 12th Canadian Conference on International Health, Ottawa, Canada, 9 November 2005.

12   WHO, *Report by the Secretariat on the Recruitment of Health Workers from the Developing World*, WHO Document EB114/5, 19 April 2004, para. 2. Also, see generally D.A. McDonald and J. Crush (eds.), *Destinations Unknown: Perspectives on the Brain Drain in Southern Africa* (Cape Town: Southern African Migration Project, 2002).

13   P. Collier et al., "Africa's Exodus: Capital Flight and the Brain Drain as Portfolio Decisions" *Journal of African Economies* 13(2): ii15-ii54.

14   A. Astor et al., "Physician migration: Views from Professionals in Colombia, Nigeria, India, Pakistan and the Philippines" *Social Science and Medicine* 61(12): 2492-2500.

15   WHO, *Human Resources for Development*, 9 January 2006, Document EB117/36. Available at: http://www.who.int/gb/ebwha/pdf_files/EB117/B117_36-en.pdf.

16   L. Chen et al., "Human Resources for Health: Overcoming the Crisis" *The Lancet* 364(9449).

17   Available at: http://news.bbc.co.uk/2/hi/africa/4337083.stm.

18   CIHI, *Planning for the Future*, op. cit., p. 25.

19   K. Mensah, M. Mackintish and L. Henry, *The 'Skills Drain' of Health Professionals from the Developing World: A Framework for Policy Formulation* (London: Medact, 2005).

20   *Ibid.*

21   *Ibid.*, p. 19.

22   B. Stilwell et al., "Developing Evidence-Based Ethical Policies on the Migration of Health Workers: Conceptual and Practical Challenges" *Human Resources for Health* 1(8). See also *McDonald and Crush*, op. cit.

23   IRIN, South Africa: "Government wakes up to flight of health workers," 14 May 2002.

24   Available at: http://manila.djh.dk/global/stories/storyReader$98.

25   Available at: http://www.queensu.ca/samp/sampresources/migrationdocuments/commentaries/2000/nurses.htm.

26   Available at: http://news.bbc.co.uk/2/hi/africa/4506269.stm.

27   D. Mafubelu, Health Attaché, Permanent Mission of South Africa, Geneva, "Using Bilateral Arrangement to Manage Migration on Health Care Workers: The Case of South Africa and the United Kingdom," Seminar on Health and Migration, 9-11 June 2004, IOM, Geneva. Available at: www.iom.int/documents/officialtxt/en/pp%5Fbilateral%5Fsafrica.pdf.

28   Available at: http://news.bbc.co.uk/2/hi/africa/4745729.stm.

29   S. Ammassari, *Migration and Development: New Strategic Outlooks and Practical Ways Forward – The Cases of Angola and Zambia* (Geneva: IOM, 2005).

30   *Ibid.*

31   *Ibid.*

32   R. Labonte et al., *Health for Some: Death, Disease and Disparity in a Globalizing Era* (Toronto: Centre for Social Justice, 2005).

33   See generally C. Gaynor, "Structural Injustice and the MDGs: A Critical Analysis of the Zambian Experience" in *Trócaire Development Review* 2005 (Maynooth: Trócaire, 2005), pp. 67-84; F. Wood et al., *Undervaluing Teachers: IMF Policies Squeeze Zambia's Education System* (Brussels: Global Campaign for Education, 2004).

34   M. Justus, Citizenship and Immigration Canada. Presentation to the Inter-Governmental Working Group on International Migration, 28 September 2005.

35   Canadian Medical Association (January 2005). "Masterfile." Available at: http://www.cma.ca/multimedia/CMA/Content_Images/Inside_cma/statistics/dem-percent4.pdf. While other literature cites slightly higher estimates, we accept those of CIHI as more definitive; in

combining records from the Hospital Medical Records Institute (HMRI), Health Canada (Health Information Division) and Statistics Canada (Health Statistics Division) together under one roof, the Institute assumes a leadership position in providing reliable health information.

36   CIHI, *Geographic Distribution of Physicians in Canada: Beyond How Many and Where* (Ottawa: CIHI, 2005).

37   IOM, "Health and Migration: Bridging the Gap," Report No. 6, IOM, Geneva 2005, p. 82.

38   Available at: http://www.cma.ca/index.cfm/ci_id/43062/la_id/1/.

39   CIHI, *Canada's Health Care Providers: 2005 Chartbook* (Ottawa: CIHI, 2005), p. 26.

40   Justus, *op. cit.*

41   CIHI, *op. cit.*, p. 27.

42   M. Bourassa Forcier et al., "Impact, Regulation and Health Policy Implications of Physician Migration in OECD Countries" *Human Resources for Health* 2(12).

43   Ibid. See also F. Mullan, "The Metrics of the Physician Brain Drain" *New England Journal of Medicine* 353(17): 1810-18.

44   See Mullan, *ibid.*

45   Bourassa Forcier, op.cit.

46   CIHI, *Planning for the Future* (Ottawa: CIHI, 2005), p. 25.

47   Mullan, *op. cit.*, p. 1815.

48   Justus, *op. cit.*

49   D. Thurber, *International Medical Graduates in Canadian Post-MD Training Programs 1990-2004* (Ottawa: CAPER, 2005), p. 3.

50   A. Hagopian et al., "The Migration of Physicians from Sub-Saharan Africa to the United States of America: Measures of the African Brain Drain" *Human Resources for Health* 2(17) (2006).

51   Canadian Post-MD Education Registry. Visit: http://www.caper.ca/docs/pdf_quickfacts_2004_2005.pdf, p. 8.

52   *Ibid.*, p. 12.

53   CIHI, *Workforce Trends of Registered Nurses in Canada, 2004* (Ottawa: CIHI, 2005), p. 46. The number of Internationally Educated Nurses (IENs), as they are now referred to generically, who have migrated to Canada seeking employment is much higher. A recent assessment of international nurse applicants seeking to practice in Canada estimated that two thirds failed to do so, potentially leaving Canada "with large numbers of underemployed or unemployed nurses" – to say nothing of the potential impact on the health systems of their source countries. See M.E. Jeans et al., *Navigating to Become a Nurse: Assessment of International Nurse Applicants Final Report* (Ottawa: Canadian Nurses Association, Ottawa, 2005). The number of IENs (registered, licensed practical and registered psychiatric) applying for registration in Canada increased from 1,792 in 1999, to 5,815 in 2002, falling slightly to 4,546 in 2003.

54   CIHI news release "Nursing Workforce Getting Older: One in Three Canadian Nurses is 50 or Older." Available at: http://secure.cihi.ca/cihiweb/dispPage.jsp?cw_page=media_14dec2004_e.

55   A fuller discussion of the negative impacts of structural adjustment loan conditions imposed by the international financial institutions (the World Bank, African Development Bank and International Monetary Fund) on African health systems is beyond the scope of this paper. For summaries, see MT Bassett et al., "Experiencing Structural Adjustment in Urban and Rural Households of Zimbabwe" in M. Turshen (ed.), *African Women's Health* (Trenton, N.J.: Africa World Press, 2000), pp. 167-91; R. Labonte et al., *Fatal Indifference: The G8, Africa and Global Health* (Cape Town: University of Cape Town Press, 2004) and A. Breman and C. Shelton, *Structural Adjustment and Health: A Literature Review of the Debate, its Role-Players and Presented Empirical Evidence.* Paper No. WG6:6, (Cambridge MA: Commission on Macroeconomics and Health, June 2001).

56   Dovlo, *op. cit.*

57   Physicians for Human Rights, *An Action Plan to Prevent Brain Drain: Building Equitable Health Systems in Africa* (Boston: Physicians for Human Rights, 2004.)

58   A study in Tanzania found the average health worker being pricked five times and being splashed nine times per year.

59   Regional Network for Equity in Health in Southern Africa (EQUINET) and Oxfam (Great Britain), *HIV/AIDS, Equity and Health Sector Personnel in Southern Africa* (Harare: EQUINET, 2003).

60   WHO, *op. cit.*, para. 3.

61   See McDonald and Crush, *op. cit*, note 12.

62   See Astor, *op. cit.*

63   McDonald and Crush, *op. cit.*

64   Mafubelu, *op. cit.*

65   Available at: https://www.mcc.ca/english/examinations/evaluating.html.

66   One survey of costs borne by foreign-trained physicians to pursue the licensing through MCCEEs found a median of 42% of annual income was spent. Most required six months of full time study, had to purchase books, and had to take the exam more than once before passing. W. Sharieff and D. Zakus, "Resource Utilization and Costs Borne by International Medical Graduates in their Pursuit for Practice License in Ontario, Canada" *Pakistan Journal of Medical Sciences* 22(2):110-115.

67   BC College of Physicians and Surgeons, *Annual Report 2005*, p. 36.

68   Available at http://www.cma.ca/index.cfm/ci_id/43062/la_id/1.htm.

69   Available at: http://www.gov.mb.ca/labour/immigrate/infocentre/4.html.

70   Available at: http://www.immigrationsask.gov.sk.ca/common_questions.htm.

71   Available at: http://www.gov.sk.ca/newsrel/releases/2003/09/16-670.html.

72   Available at: http://www.mcaws.gov.bc.ca/amip/pnp/pdf_files/program_policy/Pol%201-1%20Objectives.pdf.

73   BC College of Physicians and Surgeons, *op. cit.*

74   For information on this Department, visit: http://www.bcstats.gov.bc.ca/whowe.asp.

75   Available at: http://www.bcstats.gov.bc.ca/pubs/immig/imm051sf.pdf.

76   Available at: http://www.immigrationsask.gov.sk.ca/whats_new.htm.

77   Available at: http://sask.cbc.ca/regional/servlet/View?filename=newdocs050805.

78   Statistics from 1993 to 2003 demonstrate rising numbers of South African trained physi-
     cians working in Canada each year (with a slight dip in 2003). Canadian Institute for Health
     Information (CIHI), *Southam Medical Database.* Statistics gathered at special request of
     authors and issued by CIHI on 12 August 2005. Job adverts placed by private clinics and
     RHAs located in British Columbia, Alberta and Saskatchewan in the South African Medical
     Journal in 2004 and 2005 demonstrate Canadian actors actively seeking to recruit from
     South Africa. See, e.g., Professional Advertising section of *South African Medical Journal*
     96(3) 2006.

79   Available at: http://www.cic.gc.ca/english/monitor/issue09/05-overview.html.

80   Available at: http://www.gov.ns.ca/health/physicians/img.htm.

81   Reported on CBC News, 25 April 2002.

82   "Summit to tackle hurdles facing skilled immigrants" *Toronto Star*, 18 October 2005.

83   *Ibid.*

84   C. Rogerson, *Health Professional Recruiting in South Africa* (Southern African Migration
     Project, Migration Policy Series No 45, 2007).

85   *Ibid.*

86   *Ibid.*

87   See generally B.T.B. Chan, *From Perceived Surplus to Perceived Shortage: What Happened
     to Canada's Physician Workforce in the 1990s?* (Ottawa: CIHI, 2002), p. 1.

88   *Ibid.*

89   *Ibid.*

90   S. Lofsky et al., "The Ontario Physician Shortage 2005: Seeds of Progress, but Resource
     Crisis Deepening" Report for the Ontario Medical Association. Available at: http://www.oma.
     org/pcomm/OMR/nov/05physicianshortage.htm.

91   B.C. College of Physicians and Surgeons, op. cit., p. 36.

92   M.L. Barer and G.L. Stoddart, Towards Integrated Medical Resource Policies for Canada.
     Prepared for the Federal/Provincial/Territorial Conference of Deputy Ministers of Health, June
     1991.

93   N. Esmail and M. Walker, *How Good is Canadian Health Care? 2005 Report – An International
     Comparison of Health Care Systems* (Vancouver: The Fraser Institute, 2005).

94   OECD, *OECD Health Data 2005 – How does Canada Compare* (Paris: OECD, 2005).

95   Joint Learning Initiative, *Human Resources for Health – Overcoming the Crisis* (Cambridge: Global Health Trust, 2004).

96   Canadian Medical Association, *Who Has Seen the Winds of Change?* (Ottawa: CMA, July 2004), p. 20.

97   BC College of Physicians and Surgeons, *Annual Report 2004*, p. 32.

98   BC College of Physicians and Surgeons, *op. cit.*, p. 35.

99   A. Kazanjian, *Nursing Workforce Study: Volume V: Changes in the Nursing Workforce and Policy Implications.* (Vancouver: CHSPR, 2000). Available at: http://www.chspr.ubc.ca/hhru/pdf/hhru00-07_NWPv5.pdf.

100 Pitblado et al., *Supply and Distribution of Registered Nurses in Rural and Small Town Canada, 2000* (Ottawa: CIHI, 2002), p. 4.

101 CIHI, *Workforce Trends in Registered Nurses in Canada* (Ottawa: CIHI, 2004).

102 One estimate for nurses found approximately two thirds of foreign-trained nurses who began the process of licensure in Canada failed to complete it for a number of reasons. See M.E. Jeans, op. cit., note 35.

103 CIHI, *Planning for the Future*, op. cit., p. 25.

104 Council on Graduate Medical Education, *Summary of Fourth Report: Recommendation to Improve Access to Health Care Through Physician Workforce Reform* (Washington, D.C.: Council on Graduate Medical Education, 1994).

105 D. Blumenthal, "New Steam from an Old Cauldron – The Physician-Supply Debate" *New England Journal of Medicine* 350(17): 1780-1787.

106 P.I. Buerhaus et al., "Implications of an Aging Registered Nurse Workforce" *Journal of the American Medical Association* 283(2).

107 Chan, *op. cit.*, p. 22.

108 L. S. Valberg et al., "Planning the Future Academic Medical Centre" *Canadian Medical Association Journal* 1994 (151): 1581-87. Numerous efforts to obtain more recent estimates of physician or nurse training costs where the assumptions were explicit and testable were unsuccessful, and all inquiries led back to this particular article. An admittedly "rough" estimate for current physician training costs was provided to us by staff in Health Canada's International Health Policy and Communications Division, which came to roughly half those in the 1994 article and likely represented a shift to decentralization of medical school training, thus reducing physical infrastructure costs per student. While the estimates in this 1994 article are probably higher than would be experienced today, the gap between the costs of training in Canada, vs. upgrading of foreign-trained persons for Canadian qualification, would remain substantial.

109 Summary of Tables 17.0 and 18.0 in CIHI, *Supply, Distribution and Migration of Canadian Physicians, 2003* (Ottawa: CIHI, 2004).

110 Summarized by Stilwell et al., *op cit.*

111 C. Levitt, "The Migration of Health Care Professionals from South Africa to Canada," Paper presented at Annual Meeting of Canadian Association of African Studies (Toronto, 2002).

112   Buchan et al., "Should I Stay or Should I Go?" *Nursing Standard* 19(16).

113   Kenya apparently matches contributions to its public health systems or non-profit health NGOs made by its diaspora. Creating a charitable tax category in Canada for émigrés making similar contributions to SSA countries could provide even more incentive for remittances with public welfare gains, and could conceivably form part of bilateral/multilateral agreements discussed in this report's next section.

114   M. Gordon and J. Bueno de Mesquita, *op. cit.*

115   WHO, *op. cit.*, para. 10.

116   C. Touez, *The Impact of Remittance on Development in International Migration and the Millennium Development Goals* (New York: UNFPA, 2004), pp. 41-52 at 42.

117   *Ibid.*, p. 44.

118   Mensah et al., *op. cit.*, note 92.

119   WHO, *op. cit.*, note 12, para. 10. It suggests that one such option "could be to structure some form of direct compensation to be paid by host countries to source countries, for example as a fax or proposal of salary paid per health worker recruited."

120   A corollary to this is the argument that Canada should deduct from any calculation of the costs of HHR migration from SSA source countries its health or medical education development assistance contributions. Such calculations are technically feasible. Development assistance, however, is not a form of economic exchange but fulfillment of international obligations (e.g. under the right to health article of the International Covenant on Economic, Social and Cultural Rights) and international financing pledges.

121   For sub-specialists, the cost estimate rises to over $2 million. All calculations for all countries would have to adjust for public, versus private, investments in training.

122   C. Nullis-Kapp, "Efforts Under Way to Stem 'Brain Drain' of Doctors and Nurses" *Bulletin of the World Health Organization* 83(2): p. 84.

123   This was most frequently expressed with reference to nurses, where recruitment by agencies in source countries is often unethical in terms of charging large fees but failing to provide either promised employment or settlement support once the nurse migrates to the receiving country.

124   As noted by P. Vidot, "Commonwealth Policies on Migration of Health Professionals" at the Bellagio Conference on International Nurse Migration, July 5-10, 2005. Available at: http://www.academyhealth.org/international/nursemigration/recommendations.htm.

125   A. Picard, "MDs back $2-billion fund to fix waiting times" *Globe and Mail*, 11 August 2005.

126   P. Sullivan, "Shut out at home, Canadians flocking to Ireland Medical Schools – And to an Uncertain Future" *Canadian Medical Association Journal* 2000(162).

127   Canadian Post-MD Education Registry. at: http://www.caper.ca/docs/pdf_quickfacts_2004_2005.pdf.

128   College of Physicians and Surgeons of Ontario, "Tackling the Doctor Shortage" Members' Dialogue, May/June 2004. Available at: http://www.cpso.on.ca/Publications/Dialogue/0504/shortage.htm.

129 The average profile of a small survey of foreign-trained physicians who have emigrated to Canada and are attempting to take their MCCEEs in Ontario supports this evidence.: 43% were aged 40-49 years followed closely by 30-39 year olds. 48% had graduated before 1987 and 33% between 1987 and 1992. 86% were married and 62% had children. W. Sharieff and D. Zakus, op. cit.

130 Mensah et al., *op. cit.*

131 Reported by CNA representative at Colloquium on the Brain Drain of Health Professionals from SSA to Canada, Ottawa, 14 October 2005.

132 Mensah et al., *op. cit.*, p. 21.

133 *Ibid.*

134 It is beyond the scope of this report to detail the contentious findings and debates about these programs, apart from noting that their emphasis on privatization, cost-recovery, public sector downsizing (including "medium term expenditure ceilings" on the amount of GDP that could be spent on public services) and rapid import liberalization led to a decline in funding for, and financial barriers in access to, health care in many SSA countries. One point on which there is little disagreement is that such conditionalities were singularly health negative for Africa.

135 Bueno de Mesquita and Gordon, *op. cit.*, p. 5.

136 See Preamble to the Convention.

137 United Nations, International Conference on Population and Development, Declaration and Programme of Action of the International Conference on Population and Development , Chap. 10, para. 1. Available at: http://www.un.org/popin/icpd/conference/offeng/poa.html.

138 *Ibid.*, para. 2.

139 Barring legal refugees which Canada is required to admit according the 1951 Convention relating to the Status of Refugees.

140 Paras. 34-37.

141 Para. 39.

142 UNGA, *op. cit.*, para. 61.

143 *Ibid.*

144 *Ibid.*, paras. 38-41.

145 *Ibid.*, para. 83.

146 Bueno de Mesquita and Gordon, *op.cit.* pp. 5-6.

147 UNGA, *op. cit.*, para. 64.

148 *Ibid.*, para. 65.

149 *Ibid.*, paras. 73-81.

150 *Ibid.*, paras. 82-85.

151 *Ibid.*, para. 63.

152   Scott et al., "Brain drain or Ethical Recruitment? Solving Health Workforce Shortages with Professionals from Developing Countries" *eMJA* 180(4):174-6.

153   *Ibid.*

154   G. Hugo, "Migration policies in Australia and their Impact on Development in Countries of Origin" in *International Migration and the Millennium Development Goals* (New York: UNFPA, 2005), pp. 199-215.

155   *Ibid.*, p. 206.

156   J. Buchan et al., *International Nurse Mobility, Trends and Policy Implications* (Geneva: WHO, 2003).

157   Nullis-Kapp, *op. cit.*, p. 85.

158   Buchan et al., *op. cit.*

159   J. Ball and G. Pike, *Stepping Stones: Results from the RCN Membership Survey 2003* (London: RCN, 2004).

160   R. Hutt and J. Buchan, *Trends in London's NHS Workforce* (London: King's Fund, 2005), p. 13.

161   J. Buchan and D. Dovlo, *International Recruitment of Health Workers to the UK: A Report for DFID* (London: DFID Health Systems Resource Centre, 2004), p. 7.

162   *Ibid.*

163   *Ibid.*, p. 3.

164   Nullis-Kapp, *op. cit.*, p. 84.

165   *Ibid.*, p. 15.

166   Buchan and Dovlo, *op. cit.*, p. 11.

167   *Ibid.*

168   For more information, see http://www.medicalnewstoday.com/medicalnews.php?newsid=17499.